Praise for *Plant-Powered Beauty*

"A plant-based diet makes you beautiful on the inside, and *Plant-Powered Beauty* gives you the tools you need to make sure you're giving your skin the best on the outside."

—*Bobbi Brown*

"*Plant-Powered Beauty* speaks to my soul. It's an intelligently and beautifully written book, which will serve to both educate and inspire you to go as natural as possible with your beauty regimen. Amy and Christina encourage us to harness the power of plants for healing and healthy, glowing skin. Right up my street!"

—*Sophie Uliano,* New York Times *bestselling author of* Gorgeously Green

"This is a must-read for anyone wanting to understand the ins and outs of beauty. Amy and Christina do an incredible job clearly explaining the function of each ingredient and the benefits for each skin type. *Plant-Powered Beauty* is a brilliant guide to navigate the world of clean beauty and how to have healthy radiant skin."

—*Annie Jackson, COO of Credo Beauty*

"*Plant-Powered Beauty* reminds the reader of what I've always believed—we should not have to compromise our health for our beauty. As a comprehensive guide to natural ingredients and their importance in every aspect of our lives, this book is an invaluable resource for anyone interested in keeping their skin, the body's largest organ, healthy and radiant without using synthetic chemicals."

—*Tata Harper, cofounder of Tata Harper Skincare*

"Beauty radiates inside out! Beauty, life, and nature are all interconnected, and the pure essence of plants is vibrational, healing and nurturing us on a deeper level. Love how *Plant-Powered Beauty* taps into this and is so inspiring with the recipes for self-care and skin regimens, which will surely make us shine bright!"

—Mina Gough, development for Standard International Management and spa director at The Standard Spa, Miami

Plant-Powered

BEAUTY

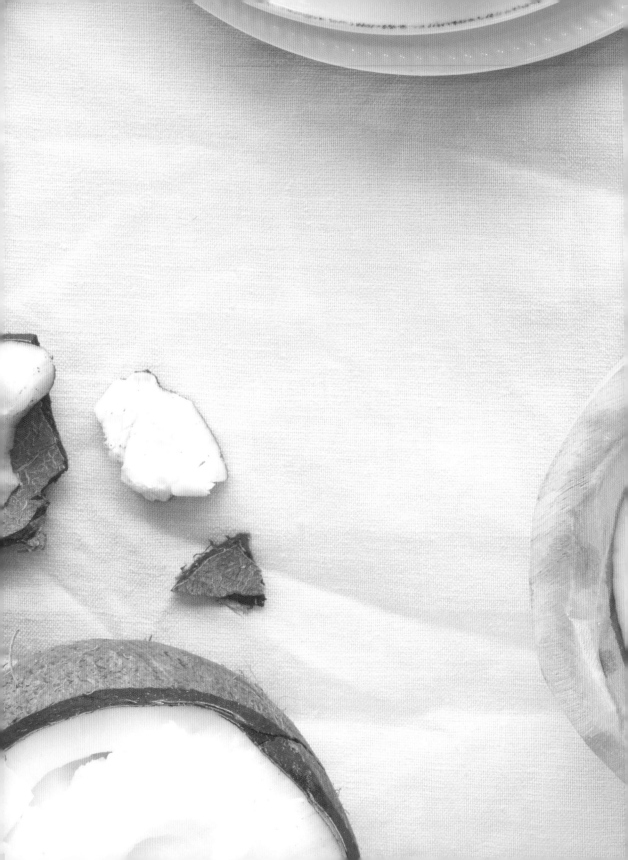

Plant-Powered
BEAUTY

The Essential Guide to Using Natural Ingredients
for Health, Wellness, and Personal Skincare
with 50-PLUS RECIPES

UPDATED EDITION
WITH NEW CBD RECIPES

AMY GALPER and CHRISTINA DAIGNEAULT

Photography by Cayla Zahoran

BenBella Books, Inc.
Dallas, TX

Cover and interior photography and Amy Galper headshot by Cayla Zahoran Photography
Christina Daigneault headshot courtesy of author

BenBella Books, Inc.
10440 N. Central Expressway, Suite 800
Dallas, TX 75231
www.benbellabooks.com
Send feedback to feedback@benbellabooks.com

BenBella is a federally registered trademark.

Printed in the United States of America
10 9 8 7 6 5 4 3 2

The Library of Congress cataloged the first edition as follows:
Names: Galper, Amy, author. | Daigneault, Christina, author.
Title: Plant-powered beauty : the essential guide to using natural ingredients for health, wellness, and
    personal skincare (with 50-plus recipes) / Amy Galper and Christina Daigneault.
Description: Dallas, TX : BenBella Books, Inc., [2018] | Includes bibliographical references and index.
Identifiers: LCCN 2017034035 | ISBN 9781944648855 (trade paper : alk. paper)
Subjects: LCSH: Beauty, Personal. | Herbal cosmetics. | Skin—Care and hygiene. | Toilet preparations.
Classification: LCC RA778 .G327 2018 | DDC 646.7/2—dc23 LC record available at https://lccn.loc.
    gov/2017034035

ISBN 9781950665679 (second edition)

Editing by Vy Tran   Cover design by Oceana
Copyediting by Jennifer Greenstein   Text design by Faceout Studio, Amanda Kreutzer
Proofreading by Amy Zarkos and Laura Cherkas   Text composition by Aaron Edmiston
Indexing by WordCo Indexing Services, Inc.   Printed by Versa Press

Distributed to the trade by Two Rivers Distribution, an Ingram brand
www.tworiversdistribution.com

Special discounts for bulk sales are available. Please contact bulkorders@benbellabooks.com.

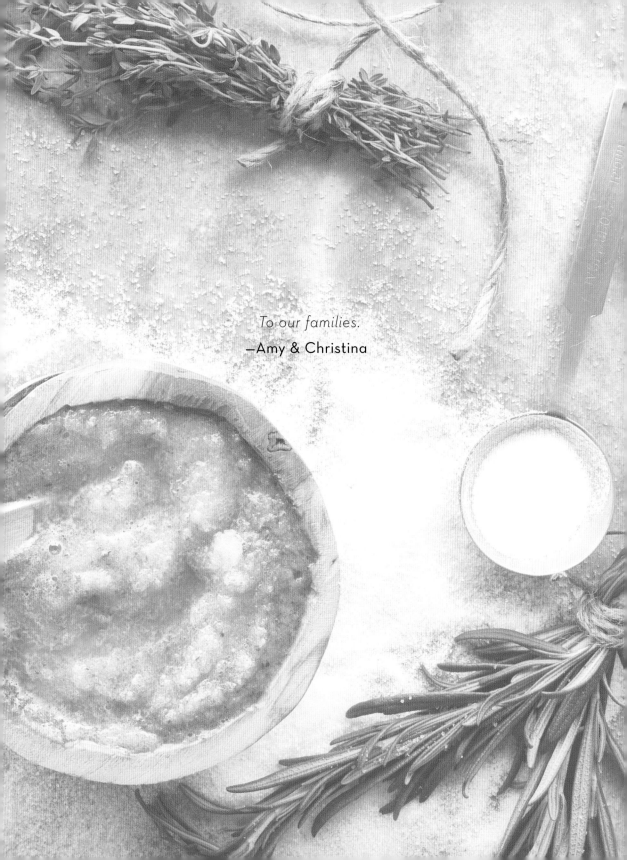

To our families.

—Amy & Christina

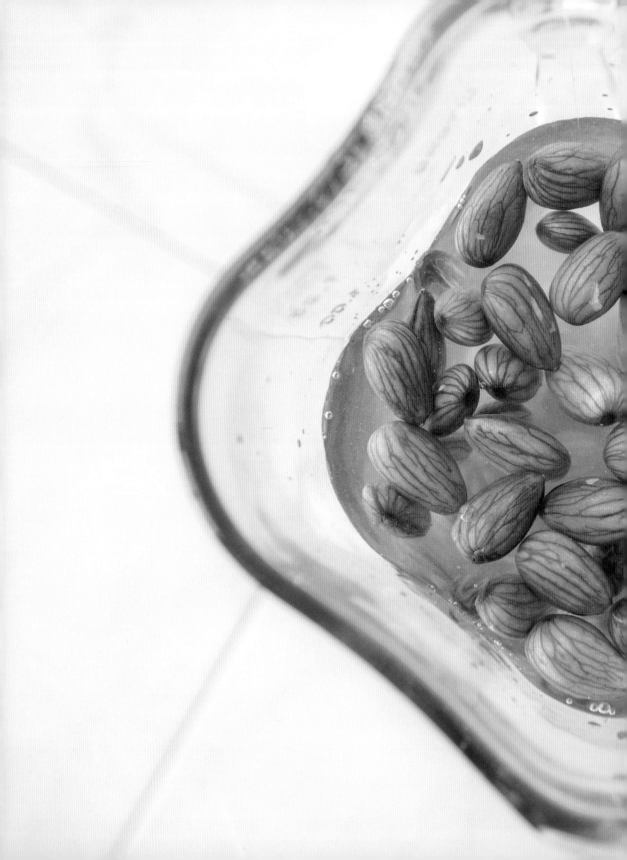

CONTENTS

Part 2 BEAUTY RECIPES

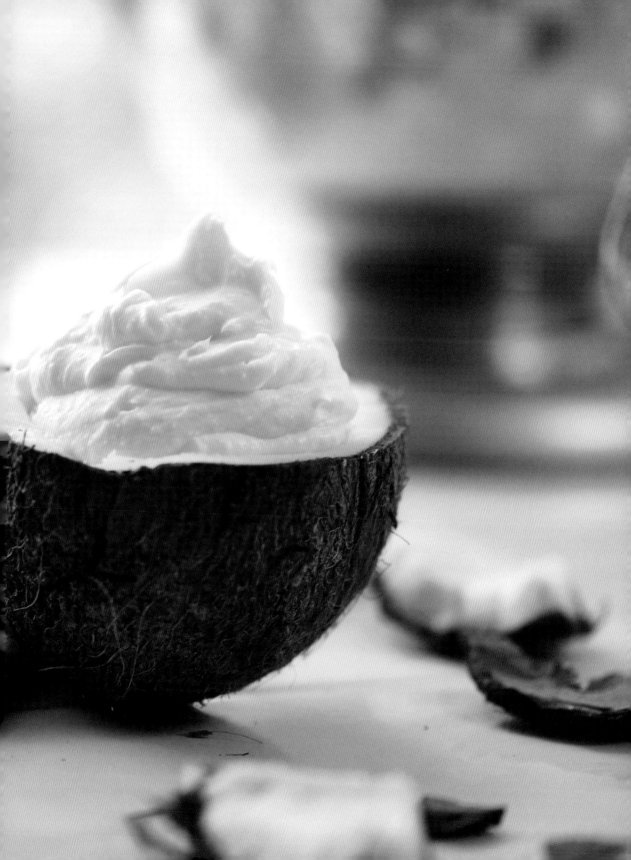

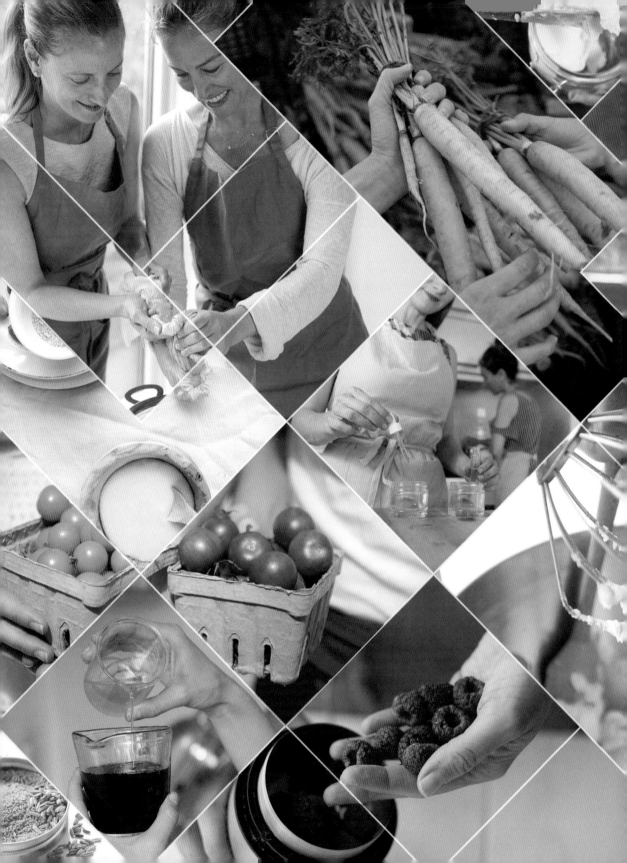

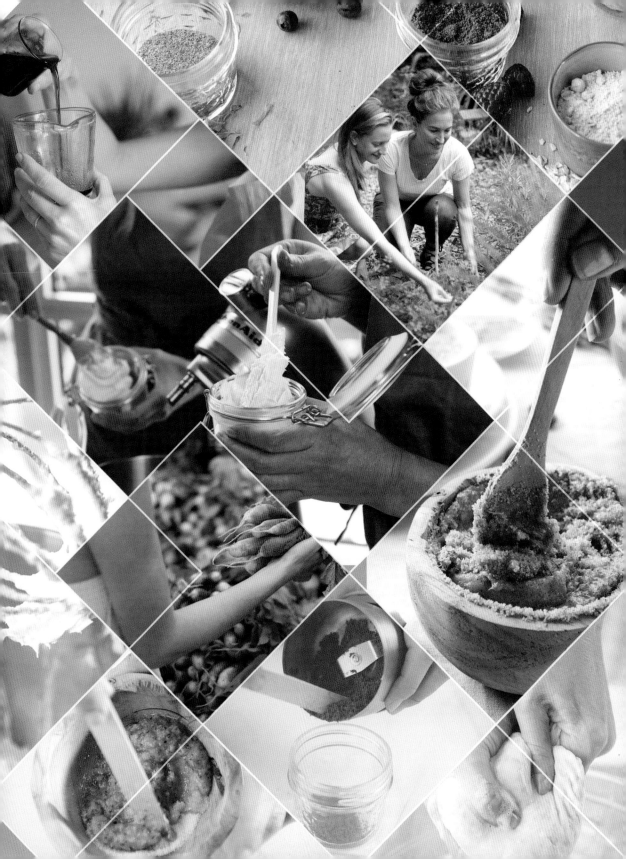

INTRODUCTION

We wrote *Plant-Powered Beauty* with a single intention—to inspire you to make your own beauty products and connect to natural ingredients in a new and exciting way. Plants have a deep impact on our day-to-day lives, and we feel confident that through the experience of smelling, touching, and blending different plant ingredients together in our easy-to-follow natural beauty recipes, you will become more aware of how plant life can support a healthy lifestyle.

As aromatherapists, we have developed a unique and dynamic formulating style that is founded on the belief that beauty is holism—meaning that the whole of beauty is made up of a healthy balance between body, mind, and spirit. We want to teach you our natural beauty blending skills so you will have alternatives to today's marketplace filled with conventional "beauty" products that contain harmful synthetic and toxic ingredients, many cleverly disguised as helpful agents of vitality. We know it can be hard to distinguish what is healthy from what is harmful, and even more challenging to find true plant-based alternatives. *Plant-Powered Beauty* will help you understand ingredients in a new light, so you can make skincare choices with confidence.

We believe that what we put on our bodies should be evaluated with the same concern we give the foods we eat. We should think about how a product is made, what ingredients it contains, how it is processed, and what its impact is on our health and the health of the environment. Our skin is our largest organ and absorbs what we put on it, and even when we rinse a product off, its ingredients get absorbed directly into our ecosystem.

Living a mindful and healthy life is the epitome of beauty, and it is our hope that *Plant-Powered Beauty* can help support your journey to this discovery.

Meet Christina . . .

I grew up on a horse farm on the North Shore of Long Island, New York, where nature was a central part of my life. I remember the lush pink hydrangeas that surrounded our colonial house at the first hint of spring and the tomato patch behind the barn where I would eat sweet fruit right off the vine in summertime. I also recall, with great clarity, the smell and taste of wild mint that grew in our pastures, the melody of crickets at night, and the excitement of watching fireflies burst into sight on late August nights.

My rural childhood helped anchor me in the world and exposed me to nature in a magical way. But it wasn't until decades later, as an adult living in an urban setting, that I was reconnected to my roots and could appreciate the generosity of plant life in a new light.

In my thirties, I became more aware of my health and the ramifications of certain food and lifestyle choices. I soon began investigating the ingredients in my personal care products and was disheartened to learn how many of them were filled with synthetic and toxic ingredients. In light of this discovery, I started to search for a better, more wholesome approach to beauty. I enrolled in a certification course at the New York Institute of Aromatherapy, where I met my brilliant coauthor, Amy, and learned about the amazing healing power of plants and the art and science of product blending. Before long, I was crafting my own beauty products with confidence and also sharing my gifts with friends and family.

What started as a curiosity about natural beauty grew into a passion, one I wish to share with others who are seeking alternatives to conventional products and would like to embrace a clean/green beauty lifestyle.

Meet Amy . . .

What we put on our skin does much more than affect our health—it does something to our spirit.

Beauty has come to mean something we have to attain outside ourselves. Women rely on nail salons, fashion magazines, dermatologists, plastic surgeons, makeup artists, and hairstylists to make them feel and look beautiful.

But what if we can do it ourselves? This book is about empowering women to make their own beauty—literally, by following our botanical beauty recipes, and more profoundly, by looking to nature to find their beauty within.

As a child I was always drawn to the woods; I spent hours during those years playing in the neighborhood ravines and counted each day until I left for summer camp, where I could canoe and sleep outside. Nature awed me, and I found deep comfort among the trees.

At twenty, a friend suggested a plant-based diet to cure a stubborn skin condition, and within a month my skin recovered. And when that happened, there was no doubt in my mind that plants held the secrets to healing.

But the real turning point came ten years later, when at thirty I was diagnosed with a mysterious autoimmune disease that threatened my kidney function and I returned to plants to guide my healing.

What happened next quickly led me to my current path, founding the New York Institute of Aromatherapy and writing this book. Since 2000, I have been on a dedicated mission to educate and advocate for conscious beauty. The journey of sharing began with my shiatsu practice and aromatherapy certification, and soon after inspired me to launch an award-winning organic body care brand. And today, I consult with a wide range of essential oil companies, natural beauty brands, and retailers, while continuing to educate people about how plants and their remarkable essential oils can raise our awareness and open our hearts.

How to Use This Book

Since we want you to become familiar with plant-powered ingredients and how they are used to make effective and beautiful skincare products, we've organized this book in a simple, straightforward way to help you make the transition from using conventional mass-produced beauty products loaded with synthetic components to beauty products powered by nature.

Part 1 offers foundational and background information; it's where we get a little theoretical and geek out, focusing on why we think it's so important to make the switch. We kick off with some simple tools to help you better understand what beauty products are actually made of, review how the skin works to absorb ingredients, and then dive deep into eleven categories of plant-powered ingredients and their healing and beautifying benefits. By the time you finish Part 1, you'll be super excited to start making your products.

Part 2 contains all our recipes. We've got you covered, literally from head to toe, with plant-powered ingredients and botanical beauty formulations. Enjoy blending treatments for your scalp, your spirit, and your feet.

The resources section gives you some food for future thought—we've shared some of our favorite resources and references so you can further your knowledge and inspire others.

Ready? Let's begin!

Part 1
NATURAL BEAUTY BASICS

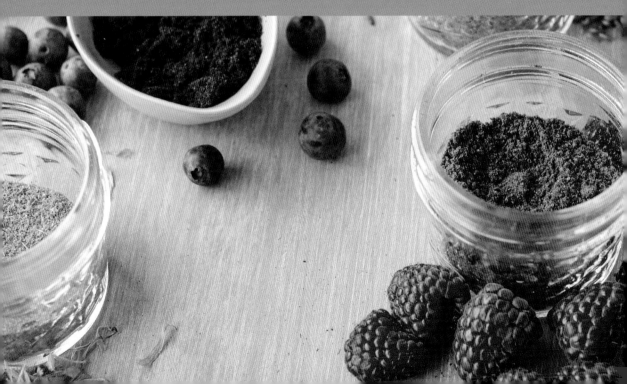

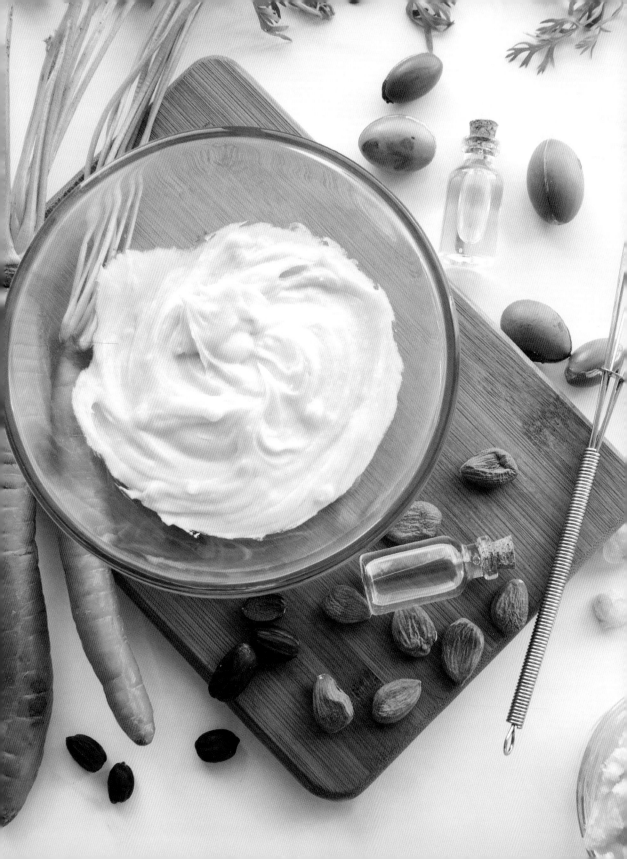

DECONSTRUCTING BEAUTY LABELS

At first glance, the majority of ingredients listed on commercially sold face, body, and skincare products look like a jumble of complicated and impossible-to-pronounce scientific names. They feel foreign and far removed from our experience. How can we connect more directly to the sources of our ingredients when the ingredients that are listed intimidate and alienate us?

When you start making your own beauty products, the world of ingredients suddenly opens up to you, and you become better equipped to decode ingredient labels found on commercially sold personal care products. What once seemed impossible to decipher becomes less intimidating—and through the clouded dust of the jargon, you can now detect a pattern and begin to interpret why specific ingredients were selected and used.

Before we share a few guidelines to help you read ingredient labels like a pro, let's make sure you understand some basics, like what an ingredient actually is and what the ingredient list (or "deck," as the industry insiders call it) reveals.

What Is an Ingredient?

An ingredient can be defined as a component of a blend, or a mixture, that contributes to the whole completed recipe. You can also think of it as a part, an element, or a constituent. In a recipe, whether for a food dish or a beauty item, an ingredient is a particular part that is added, mixed, blended, or combined to make up the whole final product.

An ingredient has two roles:

1. It has a function **in the formula**, meaning it helps make the product creamy, or sticky, or smooth, etc., and/or it has a relationship to the other ingredients in the recipe, such as the way they behave together.

2. It has a function **on the skin**, meaning it has therapeutic actions: it soothes irritation, provides moisture, softens, etc.

Ingredients come from two sources:

1. **Botanicals** are derived from plants.

2. **Synthetics** are artificially designed in a laboratory by chemists.

What the Ingredient Deck Tells Us About the Product

On a deck, ingredients are listed in descending order of concentration or prevalence.[1] In other words, the order in which the ingredients are listed reveals how much of each ingredient is actually used in the formulation, or recipe, of the product. For example, if water is listed as the first ingredient, the percentage of water is higher than that of any other ingredient listed on the label, and the product is primarily made of water. Another thing to note is what is listed last on the ingredient list; if "fragrance" is the final ingredient listed, it most likely constitutes less than 1 percent of the total formula.

By having an idea of how much of each ingredient is used, you can begin to see how the recipe is composed.

What the Order of Listed Ingredients Reveals About the Formula

A formula is basically composed of four general categories, or types, of ingredients, and each category has a very particular function within the recipe.

— The largest percentage of the recipe is composed of what many formulators and cosmetic chemists call the **base** or **foundation** ingredients.[2] This ingredient usually makes up between 65 and 80 percent of the product, and it is always listed first.

— Next are the **active** and **supporting** ingredients, which some cosmetic chemists may also refer to as *diluents* or *fillers*.[3] These ingredients often provide two different supporting activities to the recipe:

1. the actual therapeutic actions, like anti-inflammatory or skin-softening effects (such ingredients are usually easy to identify because they have names that sound like plants, botanical extracts, or specific biological compounds such as amino acids or enzymes), and

2. a textural or aesthetic function, meaning the ingredient's purpose is to combine with other ingredients to change the product's texture, consistency, or color.

This category of ingredients generally appears after the base or foundation ingredients and can constitute between 5 and 10 percent of the product.

— Following the active and supporting ingredients, we find the **functional** ingredients, which play a very specific physical (functional) role in the product (for example, exfoliant, emulsifier, or humectant). Like the active ingredients, functional ingredients may constitute anywhere from 5 to 10 percent of the formula. This category of ingredients can also sometimes share characteristics with the active and supporting ingredients, meaning an active ingredient can also be designated as a functional one. A good example of this would be soy lecithin, which acts as both a functional ingredient (it is an emulsifier) and an active ingredient (it helps make the product feel smoother).

— Listed at the very end of the ingredient deck, you will find a category of ingredients cosmetic chemists and formulators call **additives**, **adjustment agents**,[4] or **harmonizers**.[5] Their role is to pull everything together, keep the product stable, make it smell and look pretty, and so on. None of these ingredients are ever more than 2 or 3 percent of the product, and they generally include preservatives, pH balancers, colors, aromas, and other aesthetic touches.

A simple trick to help you unpack the long list of ingredient names is to try to isolate the first three to four ingredients listed, and then take note of where the first plant-sounding name appears. This will give you a general idea of what makes up the majority of the product and then reveal what the active therapeutic components may be. Everything listed that follows that first recognized active ingredient is likely to be less than 1 percent of the recipe.

A quick scan like this can immediately reveal what makes up the majority of any product. And if you see that the first three to five ingredients of a product are water and alcohol or petroleum (listed as paraffin or mineral oil), chances are there is nothing therapeutic about it.

Plant-based beauty products shouldn't be too difficult to decipher either. If they are authentic, you'll easily find that the first three to five ingredients listed are botanicals, like shea butter, beeswax, cocoa butter, almond oil, and so on. The top listing of these ingredients demonstrates that anywhere between 65 and 80 percent of what you are getting is actually from a genuine plant source and known to be therapeutic.

We've included two examples of body cream ingredient decks below, with some notes explaining how we decoded each one.

EXAMPLE A: BODY CREAM

aqua (water, eau), glycerin, isopropyl myristate, stearic acid, propylene glycol, cetyl alcohol, | fucus vesiculosus extract, hydrolyzed elastin, collagen, sodium hyaluronate, glyceryl acrylate/acrylic acid copolymer, carbomer, parfum (fragrance), sodium chloride, phenoxyethanol, potassium sorbate, methylparaben, propylparaben, sodium benzoate, triethanolamine, diazolidinyl urea, mica, CI 77891 (titanium dioxide), (red 40) CI 74.340.

Note that the first three to six ingredients (highlighted in yellow) make up the bulk percentage—we estimate about 85 percent of the product. In this case, the majority of the product is composed of water, glycerin, and a synthetically created oil, isopropyl myristate. The red line indicates the first listed botanical, and we can assume that everything that follows it will be at about a 1 percent or lower level, including the color additives, preservatives, adjustment agents, and fragrance.

EXAMPLE B: BODY CREAM

helianthus annuus (sunflower) seed oil, butyrospermum parkii (shea) fruit butter, mangifera indica (mango) seed butter, | cucurbita pepo (pumpkin) seed oil, rosa canina (rose hip) fruit oil, persea americana (avocado) fruit oil, manihot esculenta (arrowroot) root powder

This product has only genuine botanicals listed. The first three ingredients reveal what 85 percent of the product is most likely made up of: emollient-rich butters and oils. And what follows are supporting (active) botanical ingredients to increase the therapeutic actions of the product's skin-soothing properties. The arrowroot powder listed at the very end is what would be categorized as an additive; it affects the texture of the product rather than its therapeutics.

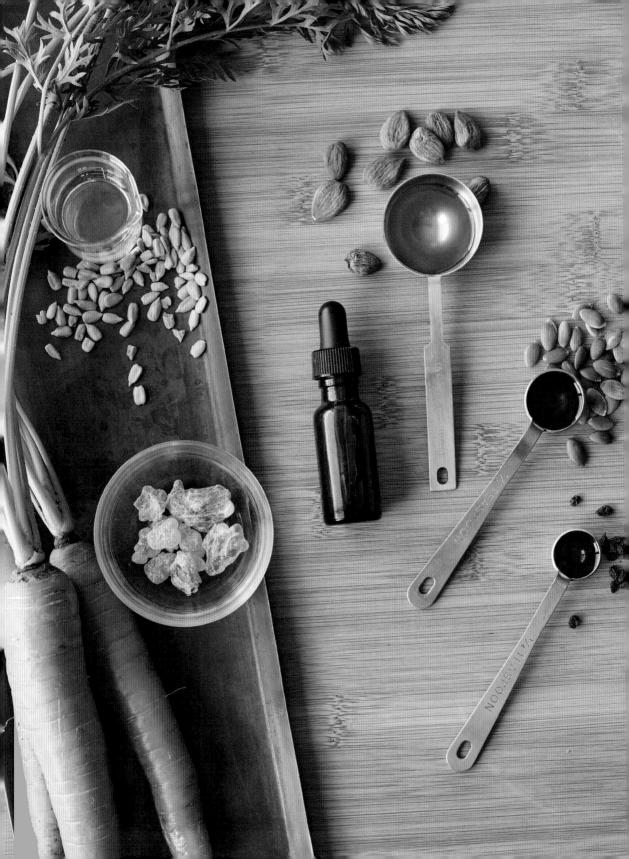

IS NATURAL THE SAME AS ORGANIC?

What's Natural?

Before we dive into our botanical beauty recipes, we thought it would be a good idea to be clear on what *natural* and *organic* actually mean when talking about beauty products.

When most people see the word *natural* on a product label, they assume that either all or some of the ingredients are natural—meaning they are not made in a laboratory by scientists. After all, the definition of *natural* from the Merriam-Webster Dictionary is "existing in nature and not made or caused by people: coming from nature; not having any extra substances or chemicals added: not containing anything artificial."[1]

Unfortunately, in today's landscape of beauty product marketing, some companies tout products as being "natural" even when there are only trace amounts of natural ingredients—or none at all. Companies can do this because, shockingly, the FDA does not regulate cosmetic product ingredients.

For our purposes, when we use the term *natural* in *Plant-Powered Beauty*, we mean it. Natural to us means ingredients that come straight from nature, and we do our homework to ensure this is the case. But we want you to be "label savvy" when sourcing ingredients or purchasing beauty products, so knowing more about the weight of this word on labels will go a long way.

How About Organic?

Thankfully, the word *organic* has a lot more weight than the word *natural*. In the United States, consumer labeling laws and USDA organic regulations require that if the word *organic* appears on a product label or in marketing material, there must be proof. In fact, the National Organic Program develops the rules and regulations of all USDA organic products and has a whole list of important checkpoints to ensure that both the ingredients and the facilities in which products are manufactured are free from toxins.[2]

Our takeaway? If you are not making your own products and are unable to trace the source of a product's ingredients, try to choose products that are certified organic by the USDA (or by EU equivalents like Ecocert, the Soil Association, and Demeter), and if you want to become more knowledgeable on the subject, check out our resources section (see page 269), where you will find suggested websites to learn more about certifications.

THE DIFFERENCE BETWEEN FOLLOWING A RECIPE AND FORMULATING ONE

Anyone can follow a recipe (and in this book, we share dozens to get you started), but our goal is to inspire you to formulate your own.

Following a recipe asks only that you follow directions, while formulating a recipe asks you to look at why and how ingredients are mixed together and tap into your knowledge, blending instincts, and creativity to develop custom products that address a particular need.

If you are baking a cake, for example, you know that you need a certain amount of flour, salt, and baking powder, measured out in specific proportions, in order to make the cake light and fluffy. And you know that if you accidentally forget to add salt, the baking powder will not react in the intended way with the flour, and the cake will likely be denser and heavier. The ratio of flour to baking powder to salt affects how the cake bakes.

The same principle works when formulating skincare recipes. If we want our healing salve to feel more ointment-like and to absorb more quickly, then we adjust and tweak the oil-to-beeswax ratio in order to get the specific consistency we are looking for.

To think like a formulator, we have to first examine each of our ingredients and understand how it behaves, not only on its own but also in combination with a wide assortment of different ingredients.

Here are a few tips to transform you from an expert recipe follower into a maverick beauty-kitchen formulator:

— **Become best friends with your ingredients.**

Get into a relationship with your ingredients and love them unconditionally. Know what they smell like, feel like, and sound like. Observe how they behave around other ingredients and materials. Discover what makes them quirky, dependable, fickle, or clingy. Take notes. Read up on their chemical constituents and study their history; get to know their every detail.

— **Mix and match.**

Start experimenting with mixing different ingredients together. Begin with mixing two, and then add a third. Play around with different proportions and observe how the ingredients change when combined.

— **Take copious notes.**

Record everything. Sometimes just adding a ¼ teaspoon more of a certain ingredient can change the entire texture or consistency of a recipe. So make sure you write down every detail of what you do. Keep in mind that the order in which you blend and combine ingredients can have an impact on the product's stability and efficacy as well.

— **Embrace trial and error.**

Make mistakes! Don't be afraid to fail miserably and make a mess. Just remember to record your findings, take photos, and document everything so you can learn from what didn't work.

HOW THE SKIN WORKS

Many of the recipes in this book go on our skin, so it is probably a good idea to learn a little about how the skin is structured and its basic functions. Having a better understanding of what makes up the different layers of our skin will provide tremendous insight as we select ingredients for our recipes, especially when we are considering specific skin types and conditions.

Our skin, also known as the integumentary system, weighs between seven and eight pounds. If it were stretched out, it would measure approximately sixteen to twenty-two square feet. Its complex and dynamic functions are essential to our overall health and wellness.[1]

The skin has seven basic functions:

1. It protects
   a. our internal organ tissue from the environment by providing a kind of cushion layer against sudden impacts, abrasion, and bumps,
   b. our bodies from dangerous UV light,
   c. our bodies from rapid evaporation of water,[2] and
   d. our bodies from environmental pathogens.
2. It regulates our temperature.
3. It performs sensory functions via nerve cells, so we can feel temperature, pressure, and pain. There has even been some recent research showing how our skin can recognize scent, through the presence of olfactory nerve cells.[3]

4.   It synthesizes vitamin D.

5.   It excretes sweat and gases.

6.   It absorbs.

7.   It temporarily stores fats, sugars, vitamins, and salts.[4]

When we are formulating our skincare recipes, we generally want to keep all these functions in mind and specifically want to think about how and what the skin absorbs and how each of the ingredients we choose can offer support to our skin's protective barrier and overall appearance.

Our skin absorbs components of whatever products we rub, massage, lather, and spray on it and then deposits what it absorbs directly into our bloodstream. There are two absorption paths that we focus on in our recipes: (1) hair follicles and (2) the lipid matrix, which can be described as the complex fatty mortar that fills the spaces in between the skin's cells. Both of these routes eventually connect with capillaries, veins, and arteries that then carry the molecules of what was absorbed all over the body.

Most skin conditions stem from a weakened or damaged lipid matrix, resulting in dry skin, acne, sensitive skin, and aging skin. When the complex cocktail of fatty acids and other substances like sterols, esters, and vitamins that compose our lipid matrix gets thrown off balance and starts to deteriorate, pathogens and microbes can enter our bodies more easily and make us ill.

Another vitally important role of our lipid matrix is to prevent our body from losing water. The official term for this is transepidermal water loss (TWL). Proper water levels in our body and our skin are also essential to maintaining our overall health.

The first few layers of our skin are made up of what's called "dead" cells, meaning they contain no water and have been completely transformed into proteins. They make up our "horny" layer and add a certain level of protection against the environment. These cells are stacked in a way that resembles a stone wall, without the mortar. The lipid matrix isn't present here because these cells need to slough off to make room for the new cells that are busy generating in the bottom layers of the skin. It's these upper layers that we want to focus on when we are making exfoliants and masks; we want to push along the process of sloughing off dead cells in order to make room for the new ones.

Sandwiched between this horny outermost layer of our skin and the layer where the cells are actually generated through mitosis (cell division) is an area of the epidermis (our skin) where the lipid matrix is rich and active. And it is this layer that we want our beautiful farm-fresh ingredients to make contact with.

Feeding the lipid matrix is really at the core of each of our recipes. We look at each ingredient, consider its unique chemical composition, and try to match it up with what we know makes up the lipid matrix, like fatty acids, vitamins, sterols, and esters. Supporting and nourishing our lipid matrix will greatly improve the overall health and appearance of our skin.

The area below our epidermis, where the lipid matrix resides, is called the dermis. And this is important for us to know because it is where collagen (the protein fibers that help give our skin shape) and elasticin (the protein fibers that support our skin elasticity) are actually synthesized and where we find our blood vessels. Our goal, then, is to try to direct our ingredients to penetrate down to this layer and ultimately make contact with our bloodstream and support and nourish the production of collagen and elasticin.

Certain skin types and conditions can often be traced directly to imbalances in our lipid matrix and in our skin microbiome. The skin microbiome is the protective film that covers the horny layer of our skin and is made up of a unique blend of our sebum (the oily substance secreted by our sebaceous glands, which are attached to our hair follicles), our sweat, and millions of microorganisms, or microbiota (bacteria), that live on the surface of our skin.

Let's look at a few different skin types and consider the function of the lipid matrix and skin microbiome and the selection of particular ingredients.

Dry, Aging, and Mature Skin

Feed the lipid matrix with oils rich in essential fatty acids (EFAs), sterols, esters, and vitamins. As we age, our lipid matrix deteriorates and loses the essential components that help prevent water loss and infections. Oils made from hemp seed or avocado can provide the fatty acids and the nutrients crucial to keeping the lipid matrix fluid and balanced, thus slowing down the formation of fine lines and wrinkles and inhibiting flaking and inflammation.

Sensitive and Reactive Skin

Avoid stripping the skin microbiome with harsh cleansers, and opt instead for oil cleansers and gentle masks. Choose oils rich in gamma-linolenic acids, like borage and evening primrose, which reduce inflammation and soothe irritation by strengthening and plumping up the lipid matrix to keep out allergens and bolster the strength of cellular membranes.

Oily Skin

It may seem counterintuitive, but one of the best ways to balance an overproduction of sebum (the oils our sebaceous glands excrete) is by actually using oil. A good choice would be either jojoba or argan. Overcleansing, even with a soap as gentle as castile soap, may strip too much of the microbiota and trigger an excess of secretion from the sebaceous glands. Honey washes and gentle white clay masks can draw in moisture without stripping natural oils, while neutralizing bacteria that may cause infections (blemishes).

Our ingredient charts (beginning on page 68) provide a wealth of information and detail on many ingredients and break down their essential fatty constituents and nutrients. The charts will help you formulate recipes for specific skin types and conditions and draw on an array of different fatty acids, nutrients, and other vital components that can heal and support the health of your skin.

PLANT EXTRACTS AND WHOLE-PLANT PARTS

As natural beauty formulators, we turn exclusively to plants for our product ingredients, carefully considering the wide spectrum of aromatic and medicinal properties unique to each one. In some instances, we may find it helpful to use the **entire plant part**. For example, in our Fresh Anti-inflammatory and Brightening Facial Mask (see page 177), we use the full strawberry as an ingredient. In other recipes we may use an **extract of a plant** to better deliver the specific constituents needed for a product's efficacy.

Your knowledge about when to use an extract (and what method of extraction is most suitable) or the whole plant part will come into focus as you learn the art and science of blending. First, let's take a look at the role of extracts and the history of their use in our world of plant-based beauty.

Plant-based beauty literally means that all the ingredients we use to formulate our recipes come directly from plants. Plants are composed of incredibly complex and amazingly rich molecular compounds that humans have learned to interact with for millennia.

The evolution and development of herbal (and modern) medicine grew out of the ways in which we interacted with plants and our observations of how they behaved within their environment. For example, the indigenous people of Australia, while living amongst the tea trees, noticed that when leaves fell into nearby waters, the waters, when bathed in, could heal wounds. This discovery made them curious and led them to understand that there was something in the tea tree plant that was somehow preventing the growth of microbes and bacteria. They wondered, if something in the tea tree prevents bacteria from growing in still waters, how can we use the tea tree to help us avoid infections?[1]

This question is at the root of what inspired early humans to figure out ways to use plants for medicine. Their interactions and experiments with plants demonstrated that certain preparations of plant material worked more effectively than others for a wide variety of conditions, and soon the practice of making medicine was in full swing.

Extraction is the process of obtaining a plant's medicinal (that is, therapeutic) constituents through various methods that are designed to get these unique components out of the plant. It is important to note that different methods of extraction yield different kinds of medicinal materials, and these varying types of materials are better suited for different beauty applications.

For example, carrot seeds, when expeller-pressed, produce a lipid-rich seed oil that is used as an emollient for skin creams, salves, and serums.[2] But when this identical seed is processed through a different method of extraction, like steam distillation, the lipid-rich components remain within the plant material, while the volatile aromatic molecules are released, vaporized, and collected in the resulting essential oil, which can be used for both physical and psychological/emotional applications.

Extractions are possible from a spectrum of plant materials, including roots, seeds, leaves, resins, wood, fruits, citrus peels, and flowers.

To help bring the concept of plant extracts into focus, so you have a better grasp of their unique characteristics for purposes of skincare formulating, we have broken down the most common approaches into nine categories of extraction methods:

1. **Steam distillation:** A process of extracting aromatic components from plant materials using an apparatus called a "still." Various plant materials, which can come from leaves, flowers, fruits, roots, seeds, wood, bark, or resins, are

collected and prepared (meaning the material is either dried, finely chopped, or ground) and then loaded into the part of the still called the retort, which, depending on the size of the still, can look like a large vat. Steam is then introduced, or pumped, through an adjacent pipe that feeds into the retort, passing through the plant material and releasing its aromatic molecules. Once the aromatic molecules are released from the plant material and make contact with the steam, they vaporize and molecularly bond with the steam, flowing through a pipe that is fastened to the top of the retort. This pipe then curves and coils and passes through a cooling area called a condenser, which transforms the steam back into its water-like state and guides it out of the still, from which it flows into a collection vessel. The essential oil, since it is not dissolvable in water, floats on top of the water (the remaining water without the essential oil is known as hydrosol) and is then siphoned off and collected separately. Since steam distillation uses only water, steam, and gentle heat, it is one of the cleanest and purest methods to extract aromatic molecules.

2. **Cold expression:** A method of extracting the aromatic molecules from the peels of various citrus fruits, like lemon, lime, yuzu, grapefruit, orange, and mandarin. In this process, the peel is removed from the fruit and then pressed under high pressure, without heat, to squeeze out and collect the essential oils. Cold expression is also considered a pure and clean method of ex-traction, resulting in an essential oil.

3. **Expeller-pressing:** A popular approach for extracting the lipids (that is, the fatty molecules) from nuts, seeds, and whole fruits, like avocado, sea buck-thorn, and olive. This process involves two steps: first the seeds, nuts, and fruits are sorted and cleaned, and then they are put in a large pressing ap-

Beauty Tip!

Be on alert that some processors may wash the nuts and seeds in high heat and/or solvent solutions to loosen the shells and break down the seed coat to make the pressing process yield higher quantities. To avoid any trace residues of solvents in your beauty products, stay away from vegetable oils that are processed with either solvents or high heat, and choose only cold-pressed oils for beauty formulating.

Beauty Tip!

We recommend selecting authentic essential oils over absolutes for your beauty recipes. Absolutes can often have trace residues of phenyl ethyl alcohol and hexane, which may absorb into the skin and disrupt the body's energetic balance.[3]

paratus that squeezes all the oils out of the raw material. Although a reputable processor will not add heat to the pressing process, it is important to note that the actual pressing motion of the machinery may cause enough friction to generate heat naturally, which can alter some of the fatty molecules present in the yield.

4. **Solvent extraction:** A process that uses a petrochemical, usually hexane, to dissolve and absorb the aromatic molecules from plant material. Unfortunately, this chemical process may consequently dull the potentially therapeutic energetic activities. The aromatic substance a solvent extraction yields is called an "absolute." This method of extraction is most often used to extract the aromatic molecules from very delicate flowers and plant materials that are not capable of withstanding the heat from the steam-distillation process. Hexane can also pull out waxes and pigments from the plant material, giving the resulting absolute a richer color and more viscous texture. Perfumers tend to use absolutes more readily than aromatherapists do because absolutes can help fix the aromatic palette, so the odor profile of the fragrance does not change over time. Solvents are also often used because they make the extraction process less labor-intensive and more cost-effective.

5. **CO2 supercritical extraction:** Also known as hyper-critical extraction, this is a process that uses liquid CO2 as a solvent to help dissolve the chemical components from aromatic and medicinal plant material for use as an ingredient. CO2 extractions may be used to scent a product (aromatic), or they can be used to extract particular therapeutic components like rosemary extract or sea buckthorn oil.

6. **Enfleurage:** A technique that uses fats, either vegetable or animal, to extract only the aromatic components of the plant material. In this process, which is usually reserved for extremely delicate flower blooms, the plant material is freshly picked and immediately placed on a layer of softened fat. The fat draws out the aromatic molecules and becomes infused with the scent. The plant material is removed, and what is left is a solid mix of scent-infused fat, which can be further diluted using alcohol or other vegetable oils.

7. **Infusion:** An extraction method in which the plant material (seeds, resins, roots, etc.) is submerged in what is called a "menstruum"—a fluid that helps dissolve particular components from the plant materials. These particular fluids are used primarily to dissolve the components in the plant material that cannot be removed by water. For example, a menstruum could be vegetable glycerin, vinegar, alcohol, or vegetable oil. The process is as follows: The plant material is usually dried and ground and then submerged in a menstruum and left alone for 2 weeks to 2 months. During this soaking

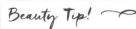

Beauty Tip!

You may find CO2 extracts sold alongside essential oils as organic and authentic aromatic materials. We love working with them, especially when we find one that fits our aromatic profile. Unlike absolutes, CO2 extracts have no concerning residues and can provide a complex scent experience—we encourage you to experiment with a few.

Beauty Tip! ⌒ℴ

If you don't want to make your own extracts and instead choose to purchase them from a verified source, make sure you ask how the infusions, tinctures, or glycerites were extracted so you can understand how all the components will combine in your recipe.

period, the menstruum dissolves the active chemical components. Once the soaking period ends, the plant material is strained, and the end product—known as an infusion, tincture, or glycerite—is the menstruum fully charged with the active chemical components of the plant.

If you decide to use an extract that you don't make yourself, make sure you know the process by which the extracts are made since the menstruum itself (that is, alcohol or olive oil) can carry with it particular skin concerns and actions. You should always ask the company from which you purchased the extract if the extract contains any added antioxidants or preservatives.

8. **Decoction:** A method in which plant material is soaked in hot water. Extractions produced by this process, also known as "teas," are prized beauty ingredients known for their gentle therapeutic properties. The soaking process allows plant materials to release their more water-soluble chemical components. These kinds of teas can be used in beauty recipes like facial masks, gels, and cleansers to enhance the recipe's healing and beautifying properties; all you need to do is blend the tea with the water or hydrosol part of the recipe.

9. **Extraction of flower essences:** The extraction of nonaromatic essences that contain only the vibrational and energetic components of the plant materials. These essences are extracted via solar or lunar energy in water. The plant material is placed gently on the surface of the water and allowed to float. It

is then left in the sunlight or the moonlight for a period of time; this process allows its vibrational and energetic components to vibrationally imprint and be memorized by the water. The plant material is removed and the water remains charged with its energetic properties. That water is then portioned off and preserved with alcohol, glycerin, or vinegar.

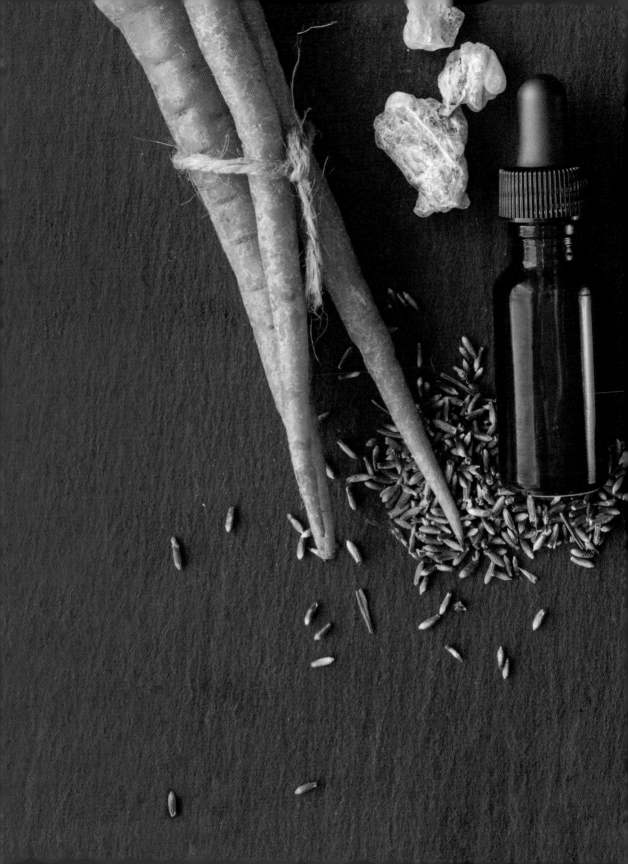

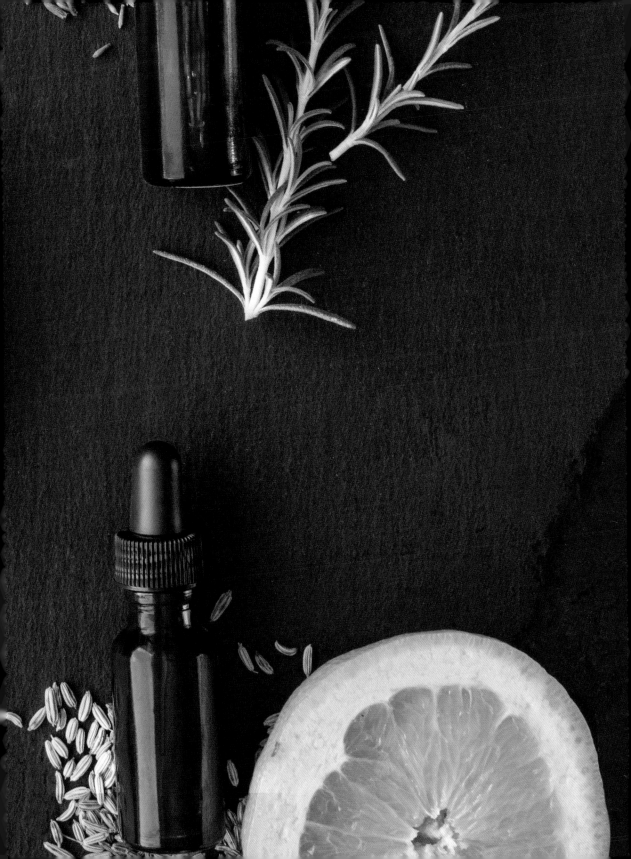

ESSENTIAL OILS AND SYNERGIES

We love essential oils. And we love blending them. That's why we have chosen to feature essential oils in almost every one of our recipes. Blending together essential oils is at the heart of what an aromatherapist does, and since we both began our journey into plant-based beauty as aromatherapists, essential oils play a key role in our formulations.

Before we begin blending essential oils together, let's review what an essential oil actually is and how the complex design of its many molecules resonates throughout the formula and works to deliver a quintessential holistic experience.

What Is an Essential Oil?

An essential oil is the distilled aromatic essence of a plant. It is made up of a complex design of many molecules (in some instances upward of a hundred) that impart both physiological actions and emotional psychospiritual experiences. As a consequence of this very unique and powerful dual function, essential oils are able to affect both the body and the mind simultaneously.

The hundreds of unique molecules that make up the whole essential oil are present at varying percentages, so when we mix different oils together, they have a remarkable ability to bond together to either increase or diminish the specific actions of the molecules that make them up.

For example, let's take a look at peppermint and rosemary essential oils. Both essential oils are made up of similar molecules with actions that help dissolve mucus in the body. By combining these two oils together in a blend, we increase their muco-lytic effect. The same goes for emotional healing and support.

As another example, mandarin essential oil is known to be uplifting. Now imagine blending it with other oils that make us feel happier. Suddenly the antidepressive actions of mandarin are greatly increased because we've blended it with other uplifting oils.

Understanding intuitively how the oils blend and smell together can take years of experience. It is a skill that requires a strong foundation in the science of aromatic medicine plus lots of practical experience actually mixing, blending, and using the oils. But we hope that by sharing our list of essential oils, along with our notes and our experiences, we can give you a jump-start on learning how essential oils work.

What Is a Synergy?

A synergy is a thoughtfully curated blend of three to five essential oils. Each oil is selected after careful consideration of its unique therapeutic action and aroma, along with an understanding that, when mixed with the others, the combined effect of the whole blend is greater than the sum of its parts.

We have chosen to include synergies in our recipes because they significantly shape the purpose and intention of each product we make. Each essential oil contributes a unique and integral action and aroma, like an anti-inflammatory or pain-relieving action or a sweet or spicy scent, to the whole synergy, and then they echo throughout the entire recipe.

Incorporating synergies into our recipes also guides the holistic experience of using the products. As aromatherapists, we understand the power of how essential oils can affect both the body and mind, and when crafting holistic plant-based skin-care, we want to make certain that the products we make feel good, smell good, and actually work.

Recipes for Essential Oil Synergies

We have designed twenty-nine unique plant-powered synergy recipes that thoughtfully combine thirty different essential oils we selected for this book. Each synergy recipe is made up of three to five essential oils, with a specific amount of drops to unleash the therapeutic and aromatic properties of the oils so they can bloom into a beneficial blend.

You will find the synergies included as ingredients in our product recipes, so we suggest referring to pages 50–53 often and premaking the synergies you intend to use most often.

We suggest mixing up essential oil blends in small, dark glass bottles and keeping them on hand for whenever you make a beauty recipe. Think of them as a kind of "back stock," or inventory, of premade blends, like a spice rack for your beauty kitchen that you can reach for at any given moment.

Feel free to mix and match the synergies with different recipes. A synergy for headache relief could also be tremendously effective for energizing tired achy feet and legs, or a synergy for sensitive skin could be lovely for soothing the itch of bug bites. Take a look at the oil chart beginning on page 54 to learn about the spectrum of therapeutic actions each essential oil offers.

HOW TO STORE YOUR SYNERGIES

You should store your synergies in small, dark 5 ml bottles that have orifice reducers—these small plastic built-in droppers reduce the amount of oxygen getting into the bottle and provide an easy way to dispense the essential oils without waste. Label and date each bottle so you can remember what is inside and when you blended it. We suggest mixing a total of at least 80 to 100 drops of your synergy to store in your bottle. The 5 ml bottles hold approximately 120 drops of essential oil.

> **Beauty Tip!**
>
> *Since our combination of essential oils includes oils that may be irritating to the skin if used individually, be careful to not get them directly on your hands, and definitely keep them away from your eyes or mucus membranes.*

DROPPING DROPS

While blending your synergies, if you find it challenging to dispense drops directly from each essential oil bottle using the orifice reducer, we suggest wiggling out the plastic piece and using a clean disposable pipette (one for each different oil) to precisely count the drops.

THOUGHTS BEFORE BLENDING

When you read through the synergy recipes, you will find the name of each essential oil followed by the number of drops. Combine all drops together in your synergy bottle, pop in the orifice reducer, and then gently shake to combine the essential oils. We have found that the synergies are most aromatic when they are given time to rest and marinate, anywhere from 2 to 24 hours, before they are used in a beauty product recipe.

CLEANSERS

Olive Oil Cleanser Essential Oil Synergy

Clary Sage	21
Marjoram	21
Mandarin	35

Foaming Honey Essential Oil Synergy

Sweet Orange	49
Rosemary	21
Fennel Seed	21

FACIAL AND BODY SCRUBS

Anti-aging Essential Oil Synergy

Carrot Seed	18
Frankincense	24
Ylang-Ylang	24
Lavender	42

Detox Essential Oil Synergy

Fennel Seed	24
Rosemary	24
Mandarin	40

Balancing Essential Oil Synergy

Geranium	27
Yuzu	27
German Chamomile	9

Cellulite-Buster Essential Oil Synergy

Fennel Seed	18
Cypress	30
Pink Grapefruit	42

Dry Skin Essential Oil Synergy

Patchouli	25
Atlas Cedarwood	40
Lavender	35

Tired Feet Essential Oil Synergy

Peppermint	30
Eucalyptus	30
Lemongrass	30

Detox Body Essential Oil Synergy

Juniper	24
Lemon	24
Ginger	24

MASKS

Deep-Cleansing Mask Essential Oil Synergy

Palmarosa	35
Geranium	21
Fennel Seed	21

Soothing Mask Essential Oil Synergy

Frankincense	28
Ylang-Ylang	28
Lavender	49

Sensitive Skin Essential Oil Synergy

German Chamomile	6
Clary Sage	18
Atlas Cedarwood	42

Hand Mask Essential Oil Synergy

Sweet Orange	35
Atlas Cedarwood	40
Ylang-Ylang	20

Foot Mask Essential Oil Synergy

Peppermint	7
Lavender	49
Eucalyptus	7
Rosemary	21

FACIAL OILS, BODY OILS, AND SERUMS

Anti-aging Essential Oil Synergy

Frankincense	20
Carrot Seed	15
Ylang-Ylang	20
Roman Chamomile	5
Petitgrain	25

Day Facial Oil for Balancing and De-stressing Skin Essential Oil Synergy

Clary Sage	15
Palmarosa	25
Geranium	15
Lavender	35

Day Facial Oil for Brightening and Circulation Essential Oil Synergy

Fennel Seed	21
Clary Sage	21
Petitgrain	35

Cuticle Oil Essential Oil Synergy

Lavender	35
Tea Tree	15
Sweet Orange	35

Healing Scalp Serum Essential Oil Synergy

Nutmeg	16
Atlas Cedarwood	32
Ylang-Ylang	16
Patchouli	20

Healthy Scalp Serum Essential Oil Synergy

Petitgrain	30
Rosemary	18
Lavender	42

Sore Muscles Massage Oil Essential Oil Synergy

Ginger	32
Marjoram	24
Clary Sage	24

Seductive Massage Essential Oil Synergy

Ylang-Ylang	28
Patchouli	35
Nutmeg	35

WELLNESS

Bug Spray Essential Oil Synergy

Cinnamon Leaf	20
Eucalyptus	20
Peppermint	20
Lemongrass	20

Mood-Lifting Essential Oil Synergy

Peppermint	6
Yuzu	24
Mandarin	30
Hemlock Spruce	30

Calming/Soothing Essential Oil Synergy

Lavender	21
Atlas Cedarwood	24
Frankincense	12
Hemlock Spruce	24

Roll-On for Headaches Essential Oil Synergy

Peppermint	5
Lavender	35
Rosemary	15
Eucalyptus	5

Blemish Gel Essential Oil Synergy

Marjoram	15
Lavender	35
Geranium	15
Thyme, Chemotype Linalool	15

Pain Relief Gel Essential Oil Synergy

Roman Chamomile	7
Peppermint	7
Lavender	49
Marjoram	21

Healthy Hand-Sanitizing Essential Oil Synergy

Lavender	18
Palmarosa	9
Frankincense	9
Lemongrass	6

ESSENTIAL OILS

	METHOD OF EXTRACTION	THERAPEUTIC ACTIONS—PHYSICAL
ATLAS CEDARWOOD /CEDRUS ATLANTICA		
PARTS USED: wood **PRICE POINT:** mid **CAN SUBSTITUTE FOR/WITH:** petitgrain, lavender, hemlock spruce **SAFETY CONCERNS:** none	steam distillation	antifungal, antiseptic, soothes irritation, antimicrobial, wound healing, affinity to breathing and respiratory balance
CARROT SEED /DAUCUS CAROTA		
PARTS USED: seeds **PRICE POINT:** high **CAN SUBSTITUTE FOR/WITH:** frankincense, lavender **SAFETY CONCERNS:** none	steam distillation	cleansing, wound healing, promotes circulation, cell regenerative
CHAMOMILE, GERMAN /MATRICARIA RECUTITA		
PARTS USED: flowers **PRICE POINT:** high **CAN SUBSTITUTE FOR/WITH:** lavender **SAFETY CONCERNS:** none	steam distillation	anti-inflammatory, antibacterial, skin soothing, wound healing, affinity for skincare
CINNAMON LEAF /CINNAMOMUM ZEYLANICUM		
PARTS USED: leaves **PRICE POINT:** high **CAN SUBSTITUTE FOR/WITH:** ginger, lemongrass **SAFETY CONCERNS:** skin irritant	steam distillation	antimicrobial, antiviral, antifungal, immune boosting, pain relieving, helps circulation
CLARY SAGE /SALVIA SCLAREA		
PARTS USED: aerial parts **PRICE POINT:** mid **CAN SUBSTITUTE FOR/WITH:** geranium, marjoram **SAFETY CONCERNS:** avoid in first trimester of pregnancy	steam distillation	antispasmodic, wound healing, anti-inflammatory, affinity to women's reproductive health

grounding, centering, strengthening, quiets thoughts

sweet, uplifting, heartwarming, nourishing, inspires manifestation

sedating, quiets mind chatter, soothes emotions, opens heart

There are two kinds of chamomile essential oils: German and Roman. German is a deep blue color and best used for inflamed skin conditions, while Roman is clear in color and is a great antispasmodic.

warming, grounding, centering, focusing, motivating

Avoid using cinnamon bark; select cinnamon leaf instead.

heart opening, emotionally sedative and balancing, soul nourishing

	METHOD OF EXTRACTION	THERAPEUTIC ACTIONS—PHYSICAL
CYPRESS /CUPRESSUS SEMPERVIRENS		
PARTS USED: *needles* **PRICE POINT:** *low* **CAN SUBSTITUTE FOR/WITH:** *juniper, hemlock spruce* **SAFETY CONCERNS:** *none*	*steam distillation*	*drying, tightens tissues, detoxifying, improves circulation, respiratory support*
EUCALYPTUS /EUCALYPTUS GLOBULUS		
PARTS USED: *leaves* **PRICE POINT:** *low* **CAN SUBSTITUTE FOR/WITH:** *peppermint, rosemary* **SAFETY CONCERNS:** *skin irritant*	*steam distillation*	*expectorant, thins mucus, pain relieving, anti-inflammatory, antimicrobial*
FENNEL SEED /FOENICULUM VULGARE		
PARTS USED: *seeds* **PRICE POINT:** *low* **CAN SUBSTITUTE FOR/WITH:** *ginger, cypress* **SAFETY CONCERNS:** *avoid in first trimester of pregnancy*	*steam distillation*	*cleansing, improves circulation, disperses stagnancy, stimulating, affinity to digestion and skincare*
FRANKINCENSE /BOSWELLIA SACRA		
PARTS USED: *resin* **PRICE POINT:** *high* **CAN SUBSTITUTE FOR/WITH:** *rosemary, lavender* **SAFETY CONCERNS:** *none*	*steam distillation*	*antimicrobial, anti-inflammatory, wound healing, cell regenerative, affinity to respiratory and central nervous systems*
GERANIUM /PELARGONIUM GRAVEOLENS		
PARTS USED: *aerial parts* **PRICE POINT:** *mid* **CAN SUBSTITUTE FOR/WITH:** *lavender* **SAFETY CONCERNS:** *none*	*steam distillation*	*antimicrobial, anti-inflammatory, cleansing, insect repellant, affinity to women's reproductive health*

uplifting, energizing, supports inner strength and
structure, focuses mind and body, helps us point
to a goal

motivates movement and decision making,   There are many different species; most can be
clears away negativity   used interchangeably.

uplifting, energizing, helps us let go, inspires our
potential, vibrant

sedative, quiets mind chatter, inspires
introspection, soul connecting

calming, balancing, relieves anxiety, opens heart   Also known as Rose Geranium.

	METHOD OF EXTRACTION	THERAPEUTIC ACTIONS— PHYSICAL
GINGER /ZINGZIBER OFFICINALE		
PARTS USED: *roots* **PRICE POINT:** *mid* **CAN SUBSTITUTE FOR/WITH:** *nutmeg, marjoram* **SAFETY CONCERNS:** *none*	*steam distillation*	*antimicrobial, antiviral, antifungal, immune boosting, antispasmodic, helps circulation, affinity to digestion*
GRAPEFRUIT /CITRUS PARADISII		
PARTS USED: *peels* **PRICE POINT:** *low* **CAN SUBSTITUTE FOR/WITH:** *orange, lemon* **SAFETY CONCERNS:** *photo-sensitizer*	*cold expression*	*drying, detoxifying, cleansing, disperses stagnancy, antiseptic, antibacterial*
HEMLOCK SPRUCE /TSUGA CANADENSIS		
PARTS USED: *needles* **PRICE POINT:** *low* **CAN SUBSTITUTE FOR/WITH:** *juniper, lavender* **SAFETY CONCERNS:** *none*	*steam distillation*	*anti-inflammatory, antibacterial, relaxes tight muscles, cleansing, expectorating, affinity to respiratory health*
JUNIPER /JUNIPERUS COMMUNIS		
PARTS USED: *needles and berries* **PRICE POINT:** *mid* **CAN SUBSTITUTE FOR/WITH:** *cypress* **SAFETY CONCERNS:** *none*	*steam distillation*	*astringent, improves circulation, disperses stagnancy, antibacterial, detoxifying*
LAVENDER /LAVANDULA ANGUSTIFOLIA		
PARTS USED: *aerial parts* **PRICE POINT:** *mid* **CAN SUBSTITUTE FOR/WITH:** *n/a* **SAFETY CONCERNS:** *none*	*steam distillation*	*antibacterial, antimicrobial, nervine, pain relieving, wound healing, affinity to all body systems*

warming, grounding, centering, sedative, balancing to emotions

Available as both fresh and dried; we prefer fresh.

uplifting, antidepressive, promotes positive thinking, helps us let go

Available as pink, red or white; we like pink for its sweeter aroma.

nurturing, quiets overactive thinking, balancing to emotions, focusing

opens mind to accept new thoughts, centering, narrows our focus

balancing, sedative, soothing emotionally, clearing and opening

	METHOD OF EXTRACTION	THERAPEUTIC ACTIONS—PHYSICAL
LEMON /CITRUS LIMON		
PARTS USED: *peels* **PRICE POINT:** *low* **CAN SUBSTITUTE FOR/WITH:** *grapefruit* **SAFETY CONCERNS:** *photo-sensitizer*	*cold expression*	*drying, antibacterial, antiseptic, skin lightening, cleansing, immune boosting*
LEMONGRASS /CYMBOPOGON CITRATUS		
PARTS USED: *grass leaves* **PRICE POINT:** *low* **CAN SUBSTITUTE FOR/WITH:** *tea tree, eucalyptus* **SAFETY CONCERNS:** *skin irritant*	*steam distillation*	*antifungal, antimicrobial, antiviral, sedative, cleansing, insect repellant*
MANDARIN /CITRUS RETICULATA		
PARTS USED: *peels* **PRICE POINT:** *mid* **CAN SUBSTITUTE FOR/WITH:** *orange, grapefruit* **SAFETY CONCERNS:** *none*	*cold expression*	*wound healing, anti-inflammatory, antiseptic, cleansing affinity to reproductive health for both men and women*
MARJORAM /ORIGANUM MAJORANA		
PARTS USED: *aerial parts* **PRICE POINT:** *mid* **CAN SUBSTITUTE FOR/WITH:** *thyme, rosemary, clary sage* **SAFETY CONCERNS:** *none*	*steam distillation*	*antispasmodic, antimicrobial, antiviral, astringent, cleansing, improves circulation, affinity to respiratory health and muscle aches*
NUTMEG /MYRISTICA FRAGRANS		
PARTS USED: *fruit* **PRICE POINT:** *mid* **CAN SUBSTITUTE FOR/WITH:** *ginger* **SAFETY CONCERNS:** *none*	*steam distillation*	*antimicrobial, antiseptic, immune protective, antispasmodic, digestive*

uplifting, energizing, antidepressive, inspires action and focus

clears mind chatter, quiets mind and nervous energy, encourages positive thinking

uplifting, antidepressive, promotes positive thinking, heart centering

sedative to nervous energy, quiets overactive mind, balances extreme emotions

warming, centering, aphrodisiac, helps us connect with deeply hidden feelings

	METHOD OF EXTRACTION	THERAPEUTIC ACTIONS—PHYSICAL
ORANGE /CITRUS SINENSIS		
PARTS USED: *peels* **PRICE POINT:** *low* **CAN SUBSTITUTE FOR/WITH:** *mandarin, grapefruit* **SAFETY CONCERNS:** *none*	*cold expression*	*anti-inflammatory, wound healing, antiseptic, antibacterial, balancing*
PALMAROSA /CYMBOPOGON MARTINII		
PARTS USED: *grass leaves* **PRICE POINT:** *mid* **CAN SUBSTITUTE FOR/WITH:** *geranium* **SAFETY CONCERNS:** *none*	*steam distillation*	*antimicrobial, cleansing, anti-inflammatory, improves circulation, wound healing, affinity to skincare*
PATCHOULI /POGOSTEMON CABLIN		
PARTS USED: *aerial parts* **PRICE POINT:** *mid* **CAN SUBSTITUTE FOR/WITH:** *tea tree* **SAFETY CONCERNS:** *none*	*steam distillation*	*antifungal, antimicrobial, anti-inflammatory, promotes circulation, affinity to skincare and immune support*
PEPPERMINT /MENTHA PIPERITA		
PARTS USED: *aerial parts* **PRICE POINT:** *low* **CAN SUBSTITUTE FOR/WITH:** *eucalyptus, rosemary* **SAFETY CONCERNS:** *skin irritant*	*steam distillation*	*expectorant, thins mucus, pain relieving, anti-inflammatory, antimicrobial*
PETITGRAIN /CITRUS AURANTIUM V. AMARA		
PARTS USED: *leaves* **PRICE POINT:** *mid* **CAN SUBSTITUTE FOR/WITH:** *atlas cedarwood* **SAFETY CONCERNS:** *none*	*steam distillation*	*anti-inflammatory, skin soothing, wound healing, cell regenerative, eases muscle tightness, affinity to skincare*

uplifting, antidepressive, promotes positive thinking, helps us let go

heart centering, mind clearing, soothes nerves, balancing

warming, relaxing, uplifting, protective, aphrodisiac, grounding

sharpens thoughts, uplifting, awakening, energizing, focusing

heartwarming and centering, balancing, promotes emotional healing

	METHOD OF EXTRACTION	THERAPEUTIC ACTIONS—PHYSICAL
ROSEMARY /ROSMARINUS OFFICINALIS		
PARTS USED: *aerial parts* **PRICE POINT:** *low* **CAN SUBSTITUTE FOR/WITH:** *thyme, marjoram, eucalyptus* **SAFETY CONCERNS:** *none*	*steam distillation*	*expectorant, thins mucus, tightens pores, cleansing, antimicrobial, pain relieving, affinity to respiratory health and skincare*
TEA TREE /MELALEUCA ALTERNIFOLIA		
PARTS USED: *leaves* **PRICE POINT:** *low* **CAN SUBSTITUTE FOR/WITH:** *eucalyptus* **SAFETY CONCERNS:** *none*	*steam distillation*	*antifungal, antimicrobial, anti-inflammatory, drying and tightening, promotes circulation, thins mucus, affinity for skincare and respiratory health*
THYME /THYMUS VULGARIS		
PARTS USED: *aerial parts* **PRICE POINT:** *mid* **CAN SUBSTITUTE FOR/WITH:** *rosemary, marjoram, eucalyptus* **SAFETY CONCERNS:** *skin irritant*	*steam distillation*	*antimicrobial, antiviral, antifungal, immune boosting, pain relieving, helps circulation*
YLANG-YLANG /CANANGA ODORATA V. GENUINA		
PARTS USED: *flowers* **PRICE POINT:** *high* **CAN SUBSTITUTE FOR/WITH:** *mandarin* **SAFETY CONCERNS:** *none*	*steam distillation*	*antimicrobial, antispasmodic, affinity to reproductive health in men and women, soothing to irritated skin and scalp*
YUZU /CITRUS JUNOS		
PARTS USED: *peels* **PRICE POINT:** *high* **CAN SUBSTITUTE FOR/WITH:** *mandarin* **SAFETY CONCERNS:** *none*	*cold expression*	*cleansing, antibacterial, increases circulation, astringent, detoxifying, clarifying*

focusing, awakening, mind clearing, uplifting, inspiring

energizing, promotes movement, uplifting, focusing, strengthens determination

gives us courage, inner strengthening, quiets mind, motivates us

aphrodisiac, euphoric, inspires love and creativity, relaxing

You can find this oil sold as fractions: I, II, III, and extra. We prefer the complete distillation.

uplifting, heart centering, energizing, clears negativity

Unique, from Japan only.

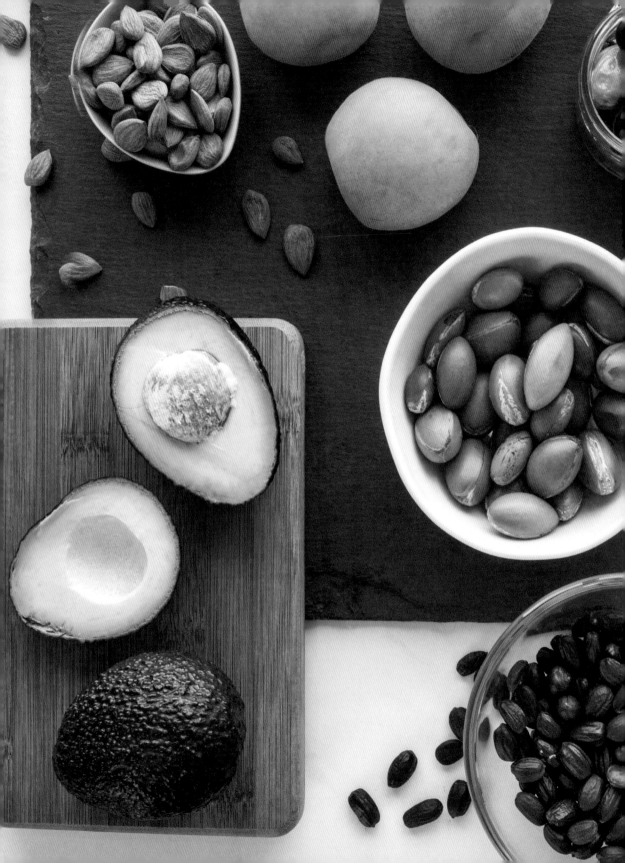

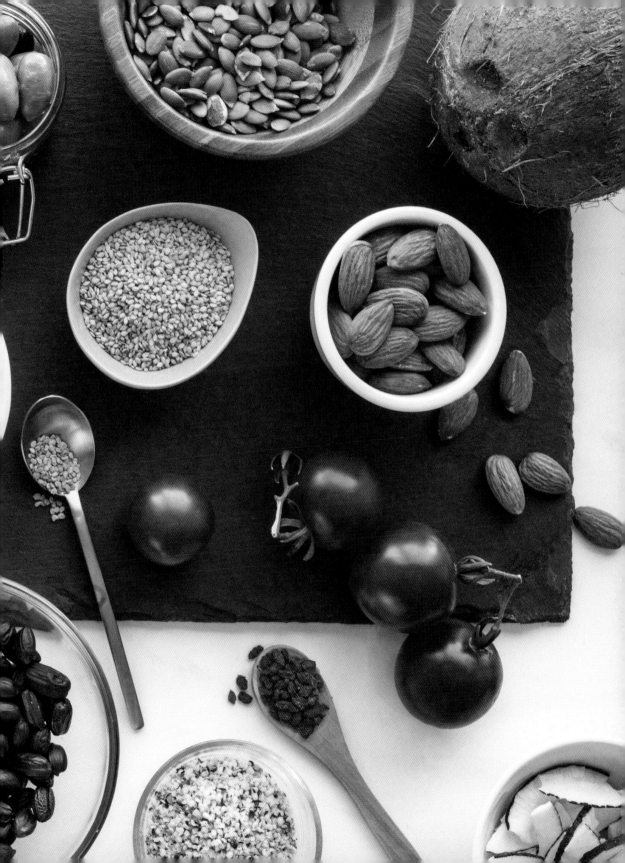

BEAUTY INGREDIENT CHARTS

We've categorized all the ingredients that we use in our plant-powered recipes into eleven charts. We hope that these simple reference charts will provide you with not only the essential go-to facts about each ingredient, so you can get to know them more intimately, but also the confidence to mix and match other recommended ingredients to create your own unique twists for many of the recipes we share.

The charts are divided into the following categories:

1. carrier oils (cold-pressed oils from nuts, seeds, and fruits)

2. herbal infusions (oils, usually olive or sunflower, in which medicinal herbs like calendula and comfrey have been soaked)

3. hydrosols (unique by-products of the steam distillation process)

4. butters (thick fatty extracts from cacao beans, mango seeds, and shea nuts)

5. waxes (from bees or plants like candelilla)

6. clays (from the earth)

7. exfoliants (including sugars and various salts that contain a rich array of minerals)

8. herbs and spices

9. flours and grains

10. fruits and vegetables

11. other ingredients (like vegetable glycerin, xanthan gum, and castile soap)

There is a wealth of information in these charts, and we hope the detailed descriptions of the ingredients and of how they are processed, along with the data on their unique therapeutic benefits, will bring you closer to experiencing how plant-powered beauty actually works.

CARRIER OILS

WHAT THEY ARE

Carrier oils are obtained from the fatty portion of a plant, such as the nut or seed. Some examples of carrier oils are almond, apricot kernel, avocado, baobab, coconut, borage, hemp seed, jojoba, olive, sesame, and sunflower.

HOW THEY ARE USED

Beauty Note!

Aromatherapists use the term carrier oils because of these oils' ability to carry the molecules of essential oils into the body.[1] But in the realm of botanical beauty formulation and organic skincare, these unique materials are better known as base oils, fixed oils, or vegetable oils.

In addition to their ability to safely dilute and solubilize the molecules of essential oils so they may be "carried" into our skin, these vegetable oils can also provide a nice source of vitamins (A, D, and E, to name a few) and a rich array of essential fatty acids, which are needed for our skin to stay healthy and hydrated.

	WHERE IT IS SOURCED	METHOD OF EXTRACTION	HOW IT IS PROCESSED
ALMOND OIL /PRUNUS DULCIS			
ALL SKIN TYPES **PARTS USED:** *seeds* **ABSORPTION RATE:** *medium* **COLOR:** *light yellow* **VISCOSITY:** *medium* **SHELF LIFE:** *1 year* **SAFETY CONCERNS:** *avoid if allergic to nuts*	*thought to be native to Central Asia; now cultivated in the US*	*cold-pressed*	*Raw nut is removed from the shell. It is cleaned, sorted, and possibly soaked in water, or a salt water solution, to remove impurities, then sun dried, or mechanically dried. The hulls then are removed, and the nuts are ground into a fine powder and pressed, yielding a "crude" unrefined oil. Refining: filtering to remove any sediment. Deodorizing: to remove aromatic components.*
APRICOT KERNEL /PRUNUS ARMENIACA L.			
ALL SKIN TYPES **PARTS USED:** *kernels* **ABSORPTION RATE:** *fast* **COLOR:** *pale to deep gold* **VISCOSITY:** *light to medium* **SHELF LIFE:** *1 year* **SAFETY CONCERNS:** *none*	*native to Iran and Manchuria; now cultivated extensively in the US and Europe*	*cold-pressed*	*Kernel is removed from the fruit, and it is cleaned, sorted, and soaked in water, or a salt water solution, to remove impurities, then sun dried, or mechanically dried. The hulls then are removed, and the nuts are ground into a fine powder and pressed, yielding a "crude" unrefined oil. Refining: filtering to remove any sediment. Deodorizing: to remove aromatic components.*

VITAMIN CONTENT	ESSENTIAL FATTY ACID CONTENT	HIGHLIGHTED FEATURES	THERAPEUTIC ACTIONS
trace amounts of fat-soluble vitamins A and E	palmitic acid: 6–8% stearic acid: 0.5–2% oleic acid: 64–82% linoleic acid: 8–28%	trace amounts of sterols and polyphenols, can offer a nice aroma when it's not deodorized, smooth feel, rich in oleic acid	emollient, skin softening, boosts immune function of skin, anti-inflammatory, healing, improves skin tone
rich in vitamin E	palmitic acid: 4–9% palmitoleic acid: 0.5–1% stearic acid: 0.5–1% oleic acid: 58–75% linoleic acid: 25–30% alpha-linolenic acid: 0.3%	great alternative for those with nut allergies; excellent for blending with other rich oils; light to touch, easily absorbed, very light feel that is richly moisturizing; similar chemical makeup to almond oil but more stable, adds great texture to facial serums	anti-inflammatory, antibacterial, antioxidant, emollient, wound healing, scar softening

	WHERE IT IS SOURCED	METHOD OF EXTRACTION	HOW IT IS PROCESSED
ARGAN /ARGANIA SPINOSA			
ALL SKIN TYPES **PARTS USED:** *kernels* **ABSORPTION RATE:** *medium to fast* **COLOR:** *light gold* **VISCOSITY:** *light to medium* **SHELF LIFE:** *1–2 years* **SAFETY CONCERNS:** *none*	*North Africa, Morocco*	*cold-pressed*	*The kernel is removed from the argan nut, which has a very hard shell and is hand pounded to open. The kernel is then mashed and squeezed to express the oil. When filtering, the oil sits so the sediment sinks to bottom and then the oil is strained and filtered.*
AVOCADO /PERSEA AMERICANA MILL.			
DRY/MATURE/ SENSITIVE SKIN **PARTS USED:** *whole fruit* **ABSORPTION RATE:** *medium* **COLOR:** *deep green* **VISCOSITY:** *medium* **SHELF LIFE:** *1 year* **SAFETY CONCERNS:** *none*	*native to the Americas, primarily Central and South*	*fresh flesh of the fruit mashed using pressure and centrifuge extraction*	*Fresh and ripe avocados are cleaned, sorted, peeled, and pitted, and the flesh is put through a masher. Next the freshly ground pulp is put into a centrifuge that spins the mash so quickly that water and oil separate out of the mash and flow into a separate vat. The oil floats on the top of the water and is separated off. Filtering comes next to remove any remaining pulp or botanical material. Sometimes manufacturers may add a little stabilizer to keep the rich green color, or some unethically may add green coloring.*

VITAMIN CONTENT	ESSENTIAL FATTY ACID CONTENT	HIGHLIGHTED FEATURES	THERAPEUTIC ACTIONS
vitamin E content exists in the crude unprocessed argan oil, also present is naturally occurring squalene	palmitic acid: 10–15% stearic acid: 5–6.5% oleic acid: 44.8–55% linoleic acid: 28–36%	the presence of squalene makes it a great skin cell regenerator and wound healer	emollient, essential fatty acids, wound healing, anti-inflammatory, antibacterial; best used for mature, aging, damaged skin, juvenile acne dry skin, and to promote healthy scar tissue
fruit contains vitamins K, C, and E and helps the body absorb fat-soluble vitamins like A, D, E, and K	palmitic acid: 7–32% palmitoleic acid: 2–13% stearic acid: 0.5–1.5% oleic acid: 36–80% linoleic acid: 6–18% alpha-linolenic acid: 0.5%	great for softening and protecting the skin; healing and soothing for dry damaged skin, and promotes skin regeneration; adds a nice softness to the skin and blends well with other oils; very nutritive because of high content of minerals; great for weakened, depleted skin	anti-inflammatory, antioxidant, wound healing, supports immune function of skin, regenerative, softening

	WHERE IT IS SOURCED	METHOD OF EXTRACTION	HOW IT IS PROCESSED

BAOBAB /ADANSONIA DIGITATA

	Africa	cold-pressed	Seeds are cleaned, separated, hulled, mashed, and squeezed. They are then filtered to allow sediment to sink to the bottom to be strained out.
ALL SKIN TYPES **PARTS USED:** *seeds* **ABSORPTION RATE:** *fast* **COLOR:** *clear to slightly golden* **VISCOSITY:** *light to medium* **SHELF LIFE:** *2–4 years* **SAFETY CONCERNS:** *none*			

BORAGE /BORAGO OFFICINALIS

	native to Mediterranean region; now present in temperate climates around the world	cold-pressed	Seeds are cleaned, separated, hulled, mashed, and squeezed. They are then filtered to remove any sediment.
ALL SKIN TYPES **PARTS USED:** *seeds* **ABSORPTION RATE:** *medium* **COLOR:** *clear* **VISCOSITY:** *medium* **SHELF LIFE:** *6–9 months* **SAFETY CONCERNS:** *none*			

CASTOR SEED /RICINUS COMMUNIS

	native to southeastern Mediterranean area, East Africa, and India	cold-pressed	Seeds are cleaned, sorted, and hulled, then put under pressure. They are then filtered to remove any sediment.
DRY/COMBINATION SKIN **PARTS USED:** *seeds* **ABSORPTION RATE:** *slow* **COLOR:** *clear* **VISCOSITY:** *thick* **SHELF LIFE:** *1–2 years* **SAFETY CONCERNS:** *none*			

VITAMIN CONTENT	ESSENTIAL FATTY ACID CONTENT	HIGHLIGHTED FEATURES	THERAPEUTIC ACTIONS
vitamins E, A, and trace of D	palmitic acid: 24.2–46% stearic acid: 2–9% oleic acid: 21–39% linoleic acid: 12–30.7% linolenic acid: 0.5–3%	anti-inflammatory and emollient, healing to damaged skin	supports collagen and elasticin, rich in EFA, fights free-radical damage, wound healing
trace amounts present	palmitic acid: 9–13% oleic acid: 14–20% linoleic acid: 34–45% gamma-linolenic acid: 25% eicosenoic acid: 3–5% erucic acid: 1–4% linolenic acid: 18–25% stearic acid: 3–5%	has a unique sterol content that means it has molecules that help cells communicate and stay strong; richest known plant source for gamma-linolenic acid	premature aging, regenerative skincare, dry or inflamed skin conditions, powerful anti-inflammatory
n/a	ricinoleic acid: 87–89.5% palmitic acid: 1–2% linoleic acid: 3–4.2% eicosanoic acid: 0.3% linolenic acid: 0.3% stearic acid: 1% oleic acid: 3–7%	nice collection of sterols that help strengthen cell membranes	anti-inflammatory, emollient, provides shine, humectant, pain relieving

	WHERE IT IS SOURCED	METHOD OF EXTRACTION	HOW IT IS PROCESSED
COCONUT /COCOS NUCIFERA			
DRY/DAMAGED SKIN **PARTS USED:** *raw fresh coconut meat* **ABSORPTION RATE:** *occlusive, slow* **COLOR:** *solid white* **VISCOSITY:** *thick* **SHELF LIFE:** *2–3 years* **SAFETY CONCERNS:** *none*	*native to the Indo-Pacific region but has since spread prolifically around the world; today, the tree/palm is mainly domesticated*	*two main processes of extraction: dry and wet. The dry method generally uses solvents; the wet process uses centrifuge and pressing*	*For extracted raw virgin coconut oil, meat can be milled, dried, mixed with water, treated with enzymes, screw pressed, and processed with the milk and the water. Coconut oil can also be sold as RBD, which means refined bleached deodorized, as well as what is called fractionated. See notes on page 103 for more of an explanation. We advise using a naturally deodorized coconut, or a raw virgin one, that is richly scented with coconut aromatic components.*
EVENING PRIMROSE /OENOTHERA BIENNIS			
DRY/COMBINATION SKIN **PARTS USED:** *seeds* **ABSORPTION RATE:** *fast* **COLOR:** *clear* **VISCOSITY:** *light to medium* **SHELF LIFE:** *6–9 months* **SAFETY CONCERNS:** *none*	*thought to have originated in Mexico and Central America*	*cold-pressed*	*cold-pressed from hulled seeds, low temperature, and low pressure since its oil is very volatile*

VITAMIN CONTENT	ESSENTIAL FATTY ACID CONTENT	HIGHLIGHTED FEATURES	THERAPEUTIC ACTIONS
vitamins A, D, and K; helps the body absorb fat-soluble vitamins more readily	caprylic acid: 6–10% capric acid: 5–10% lauric acid: 39–54% myristic acid: 15–23% palmitic acid: 6–11% stearic acid: 1–4% oleic acid: 4–11% linoleic acid: 1–2%	rich in lauric acid, a powerful antimicrobial and antiviral agent that supports our own immunity and strengthens the health of skin	emollient, antimicrobial, antioxidant, fighting free radical damage, anti-inflammatory, skin softening and strengthening, supports immunity, antiaging
very trace amounts of vitamin E, which is why it has a very short shelf life; very high in sterols, which is why it's great for cell regeneration	palmitic acid: 5.5–7% oleic acid: 14–18% linoleic acid: 70–75% gamma-linolenic acid: 9–10%	softening and deeply soothing to irritated and inflamed skin; also offering a dewy, glow-like feel that gives the experience of protection and healing	regenerative skincare, mature aging skin, psoriasis and eczema, anti-inflammatory, very healing

	WHERE IT IS SOURCED	METHOD OF EXTRACTION	HOW IT IS PROCESSED
HEMP SEED /CANNABIS SATIVA			
ALL SKIN TYPES PARTS USED: *seeds* ABSORPTION RATE: *medium* COLOR: *emerald green* VISCOSITY: *light to medium* SHELF LIFE: *6-9 months* SAFETY CONCERNS: *none*	*native to Central Asia; now widely cultivated*	*cold-pressed*	*Seeds are dried and then soaked so hull can separate, then seeds are dried again and mashed, pressed, and filtered to separate sediment.*
JOJOBA /SIMMONDSIA CHINENSIS			
ALL SKIN TYPES PARTS USED: *seeds* ABSORPTION RATE: *fast* COLOR: *golden* VISCOSITY: *medium* SHELF LIFE: *2-3 years* SAFETY CONCERNS: *none*	*Israel, southwestern US, desert regions*	*expeller-pressed*	*Seeds are often hand harvested, or mechanically gathered. It's best to harvest seeds that have ripened and fallen off the tree. Seeds are cleaned, sorted, hulled, and expeller-pressed; filtered to remove any sediment.*
OLIVE /OLEA EUROPAEA			
ALL SKIN TYPES PARTS USED: *whole fruit* ABSORPTION RATE: *medium* COLOR: *yellow to dark green* VISCOSITY: *light to medium* SHELF LIFE: *1-2 years* SAFETY CONCERNS: *none*	*originated in the Mediterranean Basin and ancient Persia*	*cold-pressed and centrifuged*	*Ripe fruits are collected either by shaking the branches or hand picking, then they are washed, sorted, and pitted. Then the flesh is ground, macerated, and pressed; the centrifuge process separates the water content from the oil.*

VITAMIN CONTENT	ESSENTIAL FATTY ACID CONTENT	HIGHLIGHTED FEATURES	THERAPEUTIC ACTIONS
high in sterols content, low in vitamin E content; particularly rich in a constituent known as wax sterols that match the chemistry of our own skin	palmitic acid: 5-12% palmitoleic acid: 0.5% oleic acid: 10-16% linolenic acid: 14-30% stearic acid: 1-4.5% alpha-linolenic acid: 25-65%	anti-inflammatory, soothes discomfort, supports skin's barrier function	dry skin, eczema, reduces water loss in skin, pain relieving, anti-inflammatory, acne, psoriasis, atopic dermatitis, regenerative, great for oily skin and to balance over production of sebum
vitamins E and B complexes, along with some minerals; high in wax esters, or sterols, which resemble in chemical structure our own sterol content in our skin	palmitic acid: 0-2% oleic acid: 10-15% eicosenoic (gadoleic) acid: 66-71% docosenoic (erucic) acid: 14-20%	a great choice for improving the overall function of the skin, boosting its immunity, and balancing its pH; extremely stable	antibacterial; emollient; wound healing; antioxidant; balancing, softening; soothing to irritations
fat-soluble vitamins E and K	oleic acid: 60-85% linoleic acid: 9-14% linolenic acid: 1%	high in sterols, polyphenols, lignans, and squalene	emollient, wound healing, cleansing, anti-inflammatory, fights free radical damage

	WHERE IT IS SOURCED	METHOD OF EXTRACTION	HOW IT IS PROCESSED
POMEGRANATE /PUNICA GRANATUM			
VERY DRY/MATURE SKIN **PARTS USED:** seeds **ABSORPTION RATE:** slow to medium **COLOR:** clear **VISCOSITY:** medium **SHELF LIFE:** 1–2 years **SAFETY CONCERNS:** none	originated in the Mediterranean basin and ancient Persia	cold-pressed	Tiny seeds are cold-pressed using nominal pressure, resulting in cooler processing temperatures; filtered to remove any sediment.
RED RASPBERRY SEED /RUBUS IDAEUS			
ALL SKIN TYPES **PARTS USED:** seeds **ABSORPTION RATE:** slow to medium **COLOR:** bright gold to reddish **VISCOSITY:** medium **SHELF LIFE:** 1–2 years **SAFETY CONCERNS:** none	US, Russia, and Eastern Europe	cold-pressed	Tiny seeds are cold-pressed using nominal pressure, resulting in cooler processing temperatures; filtered to remove any sediment.
ROSEHIP SEED /ROSA CANINA OR ROSA RUBIGINOSA			
DRY/COMBINATION SKIN **PARTS USED:** seeds **ABSORPTION RATE:** medium **COLOR:** pink to light orange **VISCOSITY:** thick **SHELF LIFE:** 6–9 months refrigerated **SAFETY CONCERNS:** none	many regions in the world	cold-pressed	cold-pressed, low temperatures as the oil is very volatile and delicate; filtered to remove sediment

VITAMIN CONTENT	ESSENTIAL FATTY ACID CONTENT	HIGHLIGHTED FEATURES	THERAPEUTIC ACTIONS
vitamins A and E	stearic acid: 1.7 % palmitic acid: 2.47% oleic acid: 4.63% linoleic acid: 9.78% linolenic acid: < 1.0% punicic acid: 66.7–80%	unique in its content of punicic acid	anti-inflammatory, cell regenerator, tissue reparative, wound healing, supports collagen and elasticin production
rich in tocopherols, vitamin E, and trace beta-carotene	palmitic acid: .9% stearic acid: 2% oleic acid: 11.7% linoleic acid: 52.1% linolenic acid: 22.2%	excellent free radical scavenger, reduces oxidative stress of the skin; low in saturated fat	rich source of polyunsaturated fats, including omega-3 fatty acids, and antioxidant activity, including tocopherols and tocotrienols; tocopherols contribute to the oil's superior free radical ion-scavenging capability and lipid support
rich in vitamin E and beta-carotene	palmitic acid: 3.33–4.97% stearic acid: trace – 0.11% oleic acid: 12.36–14% linoleic acid: 46–48.84% linolenic acid: 26–30%	tissue regeneration	regenerative skincare, premature aging, reduces hyperpigmentation, reduces appearance of age spots, softens scar tissue, tissue regenerative, wound healing

	WHERE IT IS SOURCED	METHOD OF EXTRACTION	HOW IT IS PROCESSED
SEA BUCKTHORN /HIPPOPHAE RHAMNOIDES			
DRY/COMBINATION SKIN **PARTS USED:** *berries/ seeds* **ABSORPTION RATE:** *slow* **COLOR:** *deep orange* **VISCOSITY:** *thick* **SHELF LIFE:** *1 year* **SAFETY CONCERNS:** *none*	*cold climates like Scandinavia and Canada*	*cold-pressed and CO2 extraction*	*Sea buckthorn can be extracted from either the fruit and the seeds combined or just the seeds. The fruit has a more complex collection of EFAs than the seed oil alone. This oil is also CO2 extracted from fruit and seeds and renders a very dark burnt-orange oil. Then it is filtered to remove sediment.*
SESAME /SESAMUM INDICUM			
DRY/COMBINATION SKIN **PARTS USED:** *raw hulled seeds* **ABSORPTION RATE:** *medium to fast* **COLOR:** *light yellow to gold* **VISCOSITY:** *light* **SHELF LIFE:** *1 year* **SAFETY CONCERNS:** *none*	*Middle East, Asia*	*cold-pressed*	*Seeds are hulled and then ground and pressed under pressure. They are filtered to remove sediment.*

VITAMIN CONTENT	ESSENTIAL FATTY ACID CONTENT	HIGHLIGHTED FEATURES	THERAPEUTIC ACTIONS
high in vitamin E, beta-carotene, and sterols	palmitic acid: 6–31% stearic acid: 2–4% linoleic acid: 35–40.9% alpha-linolenic acid: 20–35% palmitoleic acid: < 0.5% oleic acid: 15–28.86%	cell regenerative, soothing to damaged skin	soothes inflamed skin conditions and sun damage, wound healing, extreme dryness, mature skin, antioxidant, emollient
high in antioxidants and vitamin E	palmitic acid 8–11% oleic acid: 37–42% linoleic acid: 30–47% stearic acid: 4–6%	excellent all-purpose oil for skin soothing and healing	emollient, warming, good for dry skin, great for hair and nails

	WHERE IT IS SOURCED	METHOD OF EXTRACTION	HOW IT IS PROCESSED
SUNFLOWER /HELIANTHUS ANNUUS			
DRY/COMBINATION SKIN **PARTS USED:** *raw hulled seeds* **ABSORPTION RATE:** *medium to fast* **COLOR:** *clear to light yellow* **VISCOSITY:** *light* **SHELF LIFE:** *1–2 years* **SAFETY CONCERNS:** *none*	*US, Europe, and Asia*	*cold-pressed*	*This special process gently extracts oils, using nominal pressure, resulting in cooler processing temperatures than extrusion processes and without using any distillation, harsh chemicals, or synthetic "stripping." Then it is filtered to remove any sediment.*
TAMANU /CALOPHYLLUM INOPHYLLUM			
DRY/COMBINATION SKIN **PARTS USED:** *nuts* **ABSORPTION RATE:** *fast* **COLOR:** *deep green* **VISCOSITY:** *medium* **SHELF LIFE:** *1–2 years* **SAFETY CONCERNS:** *none*	*Polynesia*	*cold-pressed*	*The nuts are hulled, mashed, pressed, and filtered to remove any sediment.*
TOMATO SEED /SOLANUM LYCOPERSICUM			
ALL SKIN TYPES **PARTS USED:** *seeds* **ABSORPTION RATE:** *fast* **COLOR:** *light red* **VISCOSITY:** *light* **SHELF LIFE:** *1–2 years* **SAFETY CONCERNS:** *none*	*all climates worldwide*	*cold-pressed*	*This special process gently extracts oils using nominal pressure, resulting in cooler processing temperatures than extrusion processes and without using any distillation, harsh chemicals, or synthetic "stripping."*

VITAMIN CONTENT	ESSENTIAL FATTY ACID CONTENT	HIGHLIGHTED FEATURES	THERAPEUTIC ACTIONS
vitamin E	palmitic acid: 2–10% stearic acid: 1–10% oleic acid: 14–65% linoleic acid: 20–75% linolenic acid: <1.5% palmitoleic acid: < 1% arachidic acid: < 1%"	excellent all-purpose oil for skin soothing and healing; stable	emollient, anti-inflammatory
trace of vitamins but has sterols: delta-tocotrienol (236 mg/kg), stigmasterol (35.8–45.1%), and beta-sitosterol (41.1–43.1%)	palmitic acid: 11–13.7% oleic acid: 39.1–50% linoleic acid: 21.7–31.1% stearic acid: 13.4–14.3%	antimicrobial, wound healing	wound healing, anti-inflammatory, antiviral, promotes healthy scar tissue formation, good for dry/scaly skin conditions
trace of lycopene, lutein, and zeaxanthin along with phytosterols and dissolved minerals	palmitic acid: 12.9% stearic acid: 5.6% oleic acid: 20.8% linoleic acid: 48.9% linolenic acid: 1.89%	antioxidant, nutritive, protective against oxidative stress of the skin, stable	antioxidant, wound healing, protective, nourishing, anti-inflammatory, and good choice to protect against free radical damage

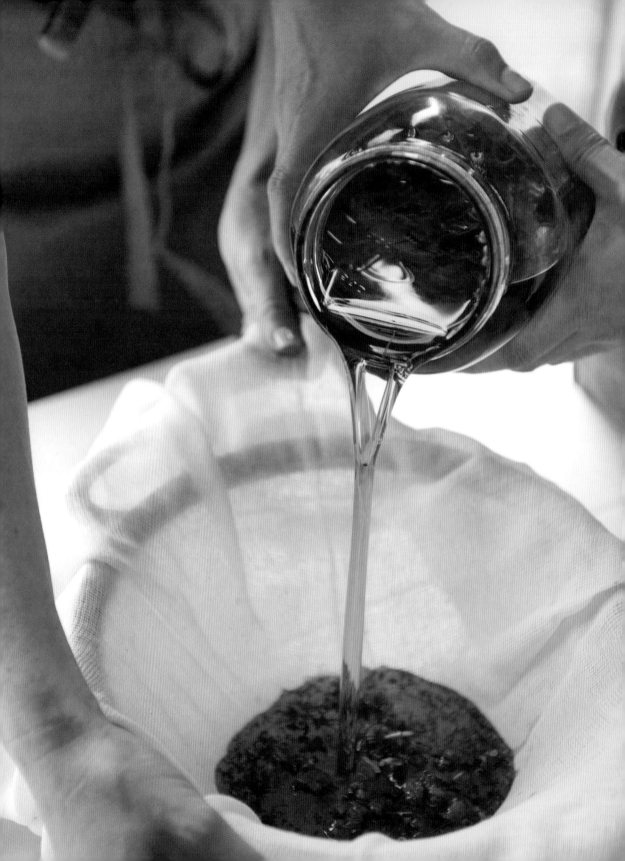

HERBAL INFUSIONS

WHAT THEY ARE

Herbal infusions are created by extracting plant properties into a carrier oil through a process called **maceration.** Maceration involves taking plant material (such as herbs, vegetables, or spices), completely drying it out and then chopping it up finely to effectively break up the cell walls, which encourages more of the plant's oil-soluble compounds to infuse and absorb into the base oil.[1] Once the plant matter is properly prepared and placed in a sterilized mason jar, the desired nut/seed oil is poured over it and sealed in an airtight container, where the blend will sit for weeks or months "extracting" the therapeutic properties of the plant material into the oil, which can then be used in a spectrum of beauty recipes.

Beauty Tip!

We encourage you to experiment with a wide variety of plant matter for your herbal infusions, but we find that olive oil, sunflower seed oil, and jojoba oil are the best bases for soaking.

HOW THEY ARE USED

Herbal infusions are wonderful beauty ingredients that can be used in place of carrier oils to enhance a recipe's therapeutic power. Whether you are formulating a facial serum, body butter, or massage blend, consider an herbal infusion with properties that complement your intention.

HERBAL INFUSIONS

	WHERE IT IS SOURCED	METHOD OF EXTRACTION

CALENDULA FLOWERS /CALENDULA OFFICINALIS

ALL SKIN TYPES
PARTS USED: dried flowers
ABSORPTION RATE: medium
COLOR: bright yellow
VISCOSITY: light to medium
SHELF LIFE: 1 year
SAFETY CONCERNS: none

Grows well in warm, temperate climates

infused in either olive or sunflower oil

COMFREY LEAVES AND ROOTS /SYMPHYTUM OFFICINALE

ALL SKIN TYPES
PARTS USED: dried roots/ leaves
ABSORPTION RATE: medium
COLOR: greenish hue
VISCOSITY: light to medium
SHELF LIFE: 1 year
SAFETY CONCERNS: none

hardy plant that is an annual; native to Europe

infused in either olive or sunflower oil

PLANTAIN LEAVES /PLANTAGO LANCEOLATA

ALL SKIN TYPES
PARTS USED: dried or fresh leaves
ABSORPTION RATE: medium
COLOR: greenish hue
VISCOSITY: light to medium
SHELF LIFE: 1 year
SAFETY CONCERNS: none

believed to have been brought to America by early colonials; considered a hardy weed that grows only where humans have disturbed the earth

infused in either olive or sunflower oil

VANILLA BEANS /VANILLA PLANIFOLIA

ALL SKIN TYPES
PARTS USED: dried bean pods
ABSORPTION RATE: medium to fast
COLOR: deep gold
VISCOSITY: light to medium
SHELF LIFE: 2-3 years
SAFETY CONCERNS: none

native to South and Central Americas; now grows in the West Indies, Madagascar, and Reunion Islands

for best results, infuse in jojoba oil

PROCESSING NOTES	HIGHLIGHTED FEATURES	THERAPEUTIC ACTIONS
Make sure flowers are dried well and maintain a rich yellow to orange color.	*rich in flavonoids that are anti-inflammatory and antioxidants*	*anti-inflammatory, antibacterial, wound healing, skin soothing, tissue repairing*
Make sure leaves and roots are dried and broken down into smaller pieces.	*contains allantoin, which is known to promote skin healing, attract moisture, stimulates cell regeneration, and that is why it is such a strong wound healer and skin soother*	*wound healing; eases sprains, torn ligaments, tendons, bruises, muscle aches, and pains; anti-inflammatory*
Make sure leaves are dried and broken down into smaller pieces.	*contains tannins and mucilage that promote and soothe wound healing and reduce swelling*	*wound healing and soothes inflammation of skin and muscles*
Use dried beans that are semi-moist and sticky.	*contains vanillin, which has been researched to have antioxidant actions along with a wide array of aromatic molecules*	*aphrodisiac, antioxidant, mood lifter, and anti-inflammatory*

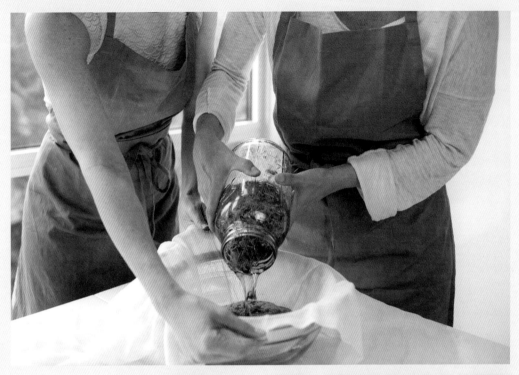

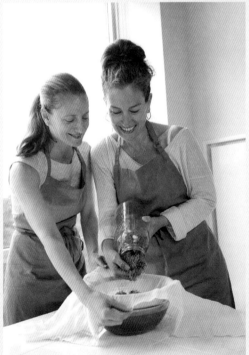

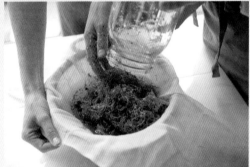

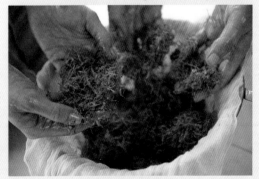

How to Make Herbal Infusions and Decant Herbal-Infused Oils

Many of our recipes include herbal-infused oils as one of the ingredients. You will find them in our recipes for face and body oils, butters, balms, treatment gels, and cleansers. Extracting the therapeutic constituents from medicinal and aromatic plants with vegetable oils is both easy and affordable and provides a varied assortment of botanicals to use in your recipes.

Infusing an oil means that we are infusing the medicinal and therapeutic properties of the plant material, which derive from its actual chemical constituents and molecules, into the oil that the plant material is soaking in. In other words, we are soaking the plant material in oil so that the therapeutic molecules are drawn out of the plant material and are able to bind with the molecules of the carrier oil. And once the plant material is removed from the carrier oil, the carrier oil is newly charged with the healing benefits of the plant.

Decanting an herbal-infused oil allows us to actually use it! We remove the plant material that has been soaking for 6 weeks to 3 months in the carrier oil by straining the oil through cheesecloth and a mesh strainer to remove any plant residue and then portion out and bottle the infused herbal oil to be used as an ingredient in a plant-powered beauty recipe.

HOW TO INFUSE AN HERBAL OIL

What you will need

° vegetable oil
° plant material of your choice, dried and chopped or ground
° glass mason jar with a tight-fitting lid
° label

1. Decide what you want to infuse and source the ingredients.

Depending on what therapeutic actions you are looking for, you will reach for different types of plant materials, ranging from a wide assortment of medicinal herbs to plant materials that are particularly aromatic, like vanilla or coffee. Once you've narrowed down the ingredients you need, we suggest finding a reliable certified organic source for the medicinal herbs you wish to infuse.

For your vegetable oil, we recommend using a certified organic cold- or expeller-pressed sunflower seed oil or olive oil. Traditionally herbalists have preferred to use only sunflower and olive oil to prepare their oil-based infusions because these two vegetable oils have been shown to be the most stable over

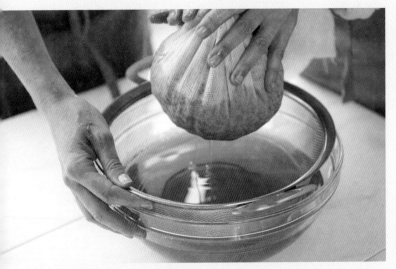
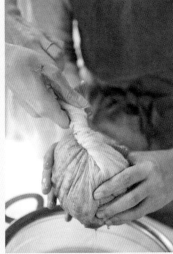

time, a characteristic due entirely to their high content of naturally occurring antioxidants, which ensure their stability throughout the infusion process.

2. Prepare the jar and botanicals.

Wash and sterilize the mason jar and its lid. If you don't have a dishwasher, we suggest boiling the jar and then wiping it down with rubbing alcohol. Make certain the jar is absolutely dry before placing any dried plant material in it.

If you are using leaves and flowering tops, lightly break up the plant materials. If you are using roots and seeds, chop and grind them roughly (this can help release the active constituents more easily into the vegetable oil).

3. Fill the mason jar.

Fill the jar loosely three-quarters of the way to the top, pour in your selected vegetable oil all the way to the rim, and cap tightly.

Label the jar with the botanical name of the plant material, the type of oil, and the date, so you can keep track of what you have made and how long it has been sitting.

Let the jar sit for 6 weeks to 3 months in an area away from direct light.

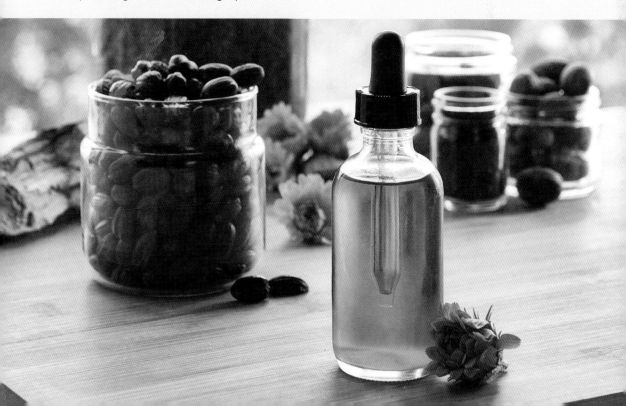

HOW TO DECANT AN HERBAL OIL

What you will need

- disposable rubber gloves
- 2 cheesecloths
- strainer
- glass measuring pitcher
- dark glass bottles with caps
- labels

1. Put on disposable gloves. Fold the first cheesecloth in half and line the bottom of a strainer. Place the cheesecloth-lined strainer over a bowl.

2. Pour all the contents of your herbal infusion (the oil and the oil-soaked plant material) into the strainer, making sure the edges of the cheesecloth don't fall into the strainer.

3. Once all the contents of your herbal infusion are emptied into the strainer, lift up the edges of the cheesecloth and bring them together as if you were about to tie the edges together.

4. Holding the edges of the cheesecloth together, twist and squeeze with your hands to wring out all the oil from the plant material into the strainer, letting the oil drip into the bowl.

5. Once it feels like the oil is completely squeezed out of the cheesecloth, lift the strainer and set aside the spent cheesecloth filled with the plant material.

6. Use a sterilized glass measuring pitcher to ladle out the herbal-infused oil into the empty bottles. If you find that some residual plant material or sediment is floating in the oil, you can strain again through the second cheesecloth and try to get the oil to be as clear of plant material as possible.

7. Cap the bottles and label them with the botanical name of the plant material, the type of oil, and the date decanted.

8. Store in a temperate area away from direct light. We recommend to use it within 1 year of decanting.

HYDROSOLS

WHAT THEY ARE

Hydrosols are the aromatic waters created during the steam distillation of plant material. They contain components of the aromatic essence of the plant, just like essential oils, but in a less concentrated form. What we love about hydrosols is their gentle, medicinal qualities, which are appropriate for a spectrum of beauty needs.

Beauty Note!

The word hydrosol literally breaks down to hydro, meaning water, and sol, meaning solution.[1] Some beauty practitioners and formulators also refer to hydrosols as hydrolates, floral waters, or distillates.[2]

HOW THEY ARE USED

Hydrosols are highly useful beauty ingredients that possess a range of beneficial properties depending on the plants from which they were created, including anti-inflammatory, soothing, antiseptic, and tissue-reparative actions. We turn to hydrosols in many of our recipes, including the spray deodorant, mouthwash, facial scrubs, gels, and facial steam. Hydrosols are also useful as stand-alone beauty companions—think toners and makeup removers. We recommend having a selection on hand in your home beauty lab.

	WHERE IT IS SOURCED	METHOD OF EXTRACTION

CALENDULA /CALENDULA OFFICINALIS

ALL SKIN TYPES PARTS USED: *blossoms* COLOR: *clear* SHELF LIFE: *1 year* SAFETY CONCERNS: *none*	*Grows well in warm, temperate climates*	*steam-distilled*

DOUGLAS FIR /PSEUDOTSUGA MENZIESII

ALL SKIN TYPES PARTS USED: *needles and twigs* COLOR: *clear* SHELF LIFE: *1 year* SAFETY CONCERNS: *none*	*native to western North America*	*steam-distilled*

GERMAN CHAMOMILE /MATRICARIA CHAMOMILLA

ALL SKIN TYPES PARTS USED: *flowers* COLOR: *clear to light yellow* SHELF LIFE: *1 year* SAFETY CONCERNS: *none*	*grows well in warm, temperate climates*	*steam-distilled*

LAVENDER /LAVANDULA ANGUSTIFOLIA

ALL SKIN TYPES PARTS USED: *flowering tops* COLOR: *clear* SHELF LIFE: *1 year* SAFETY CONCERNS: *none*	*native to Europe, Africa, and Asia*	*steam-distilled*

LEMON BALM /MELISSA OFFICINALIS

COMBINATION/OILY SKIN PARTS USED: *top leaves* COLOR: *clear* SHELF LIFE: *1 year* SAFETY CONCERNS: *none*	*native to South Central Asia, Iran, and Europe*	*steam-distilled*

HIGHLIGHTED FEATURES	THERAPEUTIC ACTIONS
wound healing, tissue repair	antibacterial, antimicrobial, anti-inflammatory, and analgesic; especially soothing for dry, itchy, irritated, damaged, or problem skin
astringent, antiseptic	uplifting, refreshing, gently energizing; rejuvenating, purifying, and tonifying
anti-inflammatory	antibacterial, anti-inflammatory, and calming, while supporting soothing relief for reactive skin; great for sensitive skin and inflammations like acne
anti-inflammatory, antibacterial, and sedating	anti-inflammatory, soothing, toning, antiseptic, healing, astringent, sedative
antimicrobial, clarifying	antiviral, anti-inflammatory, soothing to acne breakouts, rashes, insect bites, most skin irritations, sunburn, eczema, and even herpes sores

	WHERE IT IS SOURCED	METHOD OF EXTRACTION

NEROLI /CITRUS AURANTIUM

ALL SKIN TYPES
PARTS USED: *blossoms*
COLOR: *clear*
SHELF LIFE: *1 year*
SAFETY CONCERNS: *none*

native to southeast Asia, but has spread around the world — steam-distilled

PEPPERMINT /MENTHA PIPERITA

ALL SKIN TYPES
PARTS USED: *flowering plant*
COLOR: *clear*
SHELF LIFE: *1 year*
SAFETY CONCERNS: *none*

native to Europe and the Middle East — steam-distilled

ROSE /ROSA DAMASCENA

COMBINATION/OILY SKIN
PARTS USED: *flower petals*
COLOR: *clear*
SHELF LIFE: *1 year*
SAFETY CONCERNS: *none*

native to Middle East and Central Asia, now primarily cultivated in Eastern Europe — steam-distilled

ROSE GERANIUM /PELARGONIUM GRAVEOLENS

ALL SKIN TYPES
PARTS USED: *flowers and top leaves*
COLOR: *clear*
SHELF LIFE: *1 year*
SAFETY CONCERNS: *none*

native to South Africa — steam-distilled

ROSEMARY /ROSMARINUS OFFICINALIS

COMBINATION/OILY SKIN
PARTS USED: *leaves*
COLOR: *clear*
SHELF LIFE: *1 year*
SAFETY CONCERNS: *none"*

native to Mediterranean region — steam-distilled

HIGHLIGHTED FEATURES	THERAPEUTIC ACTIONS
anti-anxiety and balancing for emotions	emotionally uplifting while balancing, regenerative, astringent, calming, and soothing for the skin
cooling, pain relieving	cleansing and clearing, supports clear thinking, awakening, antibacterial, antiseptic, anti-inflammatory, reduces pain, astringent, tonifying for skin; may encourage increase in circulation
emotionally soothing and skin tonifying	moisturizing, balancing, calming, sedating, relaxing, appropriate for wide range of skin irritations and inflammations; can help soothe grief, depression, stress, and anxiety
antibacterial, antimicrobial, balancing	especially helpful for breakouts, insect bites, bruises, burns, cuts, most skin irritations, poor circulation, and stress
astringent, cleansing	stimulating, uplifting, energizing, antibacterial, and antiseptic

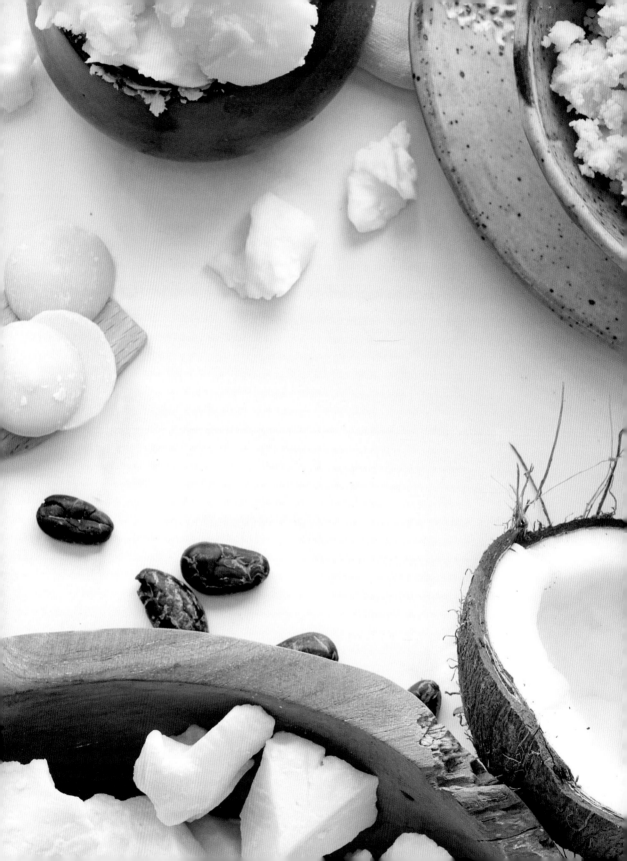

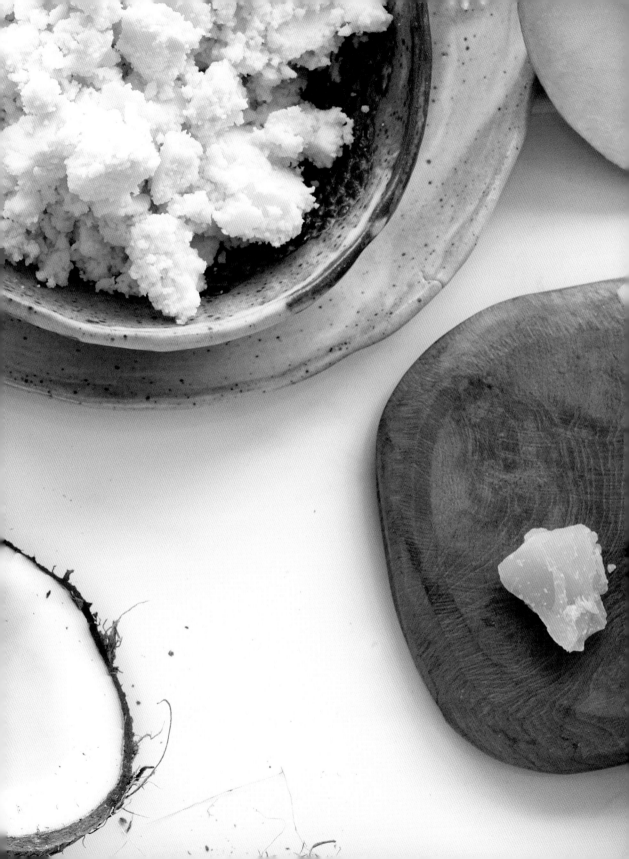

BUTTERS

WHAT THEY ARE

Butters are the fats extracted from the nuts/kernels/seeds of plants. They feel luxurious, melt on contact, and are deeply hydrating.

HOW THEY ARE USED

Some butters can be used directly on the skin, while others are best when combined with carrier oils. You will notice we use butters in many of our recipes, including our lip balm and shea butter face cream. In general, butters are great as emollients, meaning they are exceptional at softening dry, scaly skin buildup; they support the complex mix of natural fats that help glue our skin cells together and carry necessary nutrients, like vitamins, antioxidants, and fatty acids, into the layers of the epidermis.

Refined, Deodorized, and Bleached: Important Concepts to Understand About Butters

When purchasing raw butters to use as ingredients in your botanical beauty products, you may run across specific terminology used to describe how they are extracted and processed, along with other details that point to their purity and quality. This information is usually found in the product description, shared by the supplier, or provided in the butter's data profile, as well as on the label.

The most common terminology you will find to describe the purity and quality of a butter is whether it is "unrefined" (or "raw") or, on the other hand, "RBD" (which stands for refined, bleached, and deodorized). RBD means that after the butter has been extracted, it has been put through additional processes to remove (1) particulate matter and impurities, (2) any residual plant odors, (3) any residual color pigments, and (4) certain chemical constituents that consumers may find undesirable, like the heavy fatty molecules in coconut oil.[1]

For those of us using butters and vegetable oils for botanical beauty recipes, it's good practice to understand how these different methods of processing affect the ingredient's quality:

— **Refined:** A citric acid solution is used to draw out chemical components of the butter that may cause the butter to spoil quickly; this type of refining may in some instances help stabilize the butter for a longer shelf life.[2]

Another kind of refining process involves pouring the melted butter (or oil) through a sieve to separate out any minute particulates.[3]

— **Deodorized:** The volatile aromatic components of the butter are removed through a steam distillation process.[4]

— **Bleached:** The color pigments are removed using clays to draw out and absorb pigments and waxes.[5]

The best practice, however, is to look for minimally processed butters and oils that still have their genuine colors and odors intact, which means many of their health-benefiting properties are still present.

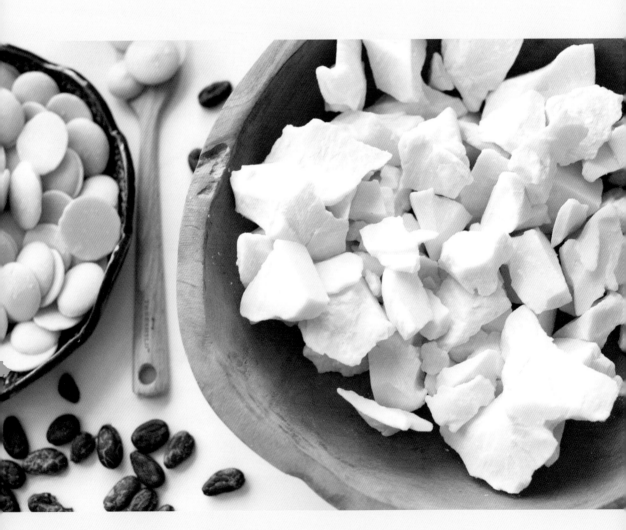

WAXES

WHAT THEY ARE

Waxes come in two varieties: beeswax and plant wax. Beeswax is a natural secretion from the honeybee, which feeds on botanicals, and plant wax is found on certain plant leaves. We primarily use beeswax in our recipes since we find it offers the best consistency, but we are mindful that vegans may opt for a plant variety, such as carnauba or candelilla.

HOW THEY ARE USED

Waxes help build thickness and create texture in products. They also support emulsification, allowing two liquids (such as oil and water) that normally can't be mixed to come together. For example, adding beeswax to a lip balm or lotion bar helps the product hold its shape while providing a harder texture.

Beauty Tip!

Waxes should always be melted at very low temperatures first, before adding butters or oils. You may discover that adding vegetable oils or butters to melted waxes causes the wax to slightly harden. If this happens, don't worry. Just continue to stir slowly over low heat until all ingredients are well blended.

Different waxes offer surprisingly different textures: beeswax is softer and stickier in feeling, while candelilla wax is shinier and much harder—meaning you would probably use 50 percent less if you plan to substitute it for beeswax.

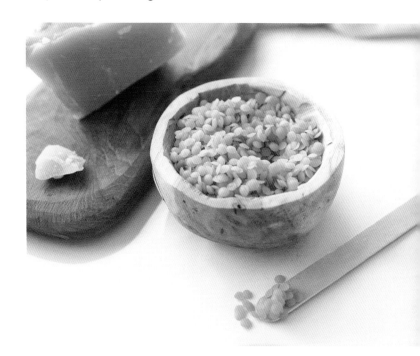

BUTTERS AND WAXES

	WHERE IT IS SOURCED	METHOD OF EXTRACTION
COCOA BUTTER /THEOBROMA CACAO		
ALL SKIN TYPES PARTS USED: *seeds* COLOR: *white to ivory* SHELF LIFE: *3 years* SAFETY CONCERNS: *none*	*West Africa and South America*	*cold-pressed from the dried and fermented cacoa bean*
MANGO BUTTER /MANGIFERA INDICA		
ALL SKIN TYPES PARTS USED: *kernels* COLOR: *cream to ivory* SHELF LIFE: *2-3 years* SAFETY CONCERNS: *none*	*tropical climates around the world*	*pressed from the dried roasted pit/stone*
SHEA BUTTER /BUTYROSPERMUM PARKII		
ALL SKIN TYPES PARTS USED: *seeds* COLOR: *cream to slightly yellow* SHELF LIFE: *1 year (raw); 2-3 years (RBD)* SAFETY CONCERNS: *none*	*West Africa*	*cold-pressed from the boiled and mashed nuts*
BEESWAX /CERA ALBA		
ALL SKIN TYPES PARTS USED: *natural secretion of honeybees* COLOR: *light yellow to medium brown* SHELF LIFE: *indefinite* SAFETY CONCERNS: *none*	*worldwide*	*collected from hives and filtered to remove impurities*

HOW IT IS PROCESSED	HIGHLIGHTED FEATURES	THERAPEUTIC ACTIONS
by-product of processing cacao beans for chocolate, it is the fat that has separated from the bean; raw cacoa butter has intense aroma of chocolate; RBD the scent of chocolate is greatly diminished	rich in essential fatty acids	antioxidant, anti-inflammatory, nourishing, soothing, hydrating, moisturizing
First the fruit stone is washed, cleaned, and dried, then it is roasted to remove the hull. The kernels are then removed and chopped or mashed and then put through a hydraulic press.	rich in vitamins A and E, antioxidant	moisturizing, cell regenerative, nourishing, soothing, protects dry and damaged skin, lips, and hair; helps shield against harmful UV rays
shea nuts are first sorted and cleaned, then ground, mashed, and boiled so the fats separate	rich in vitamins A and E	moisturizing, anti-inflammatory, helps with dry skin and systemic skin conditions
melted down and then poured through a filter	rich in vitamin A, antioxidant	antioxidant, anti-inflammatory, moisturizing, wound healing

	WHERE IT IS SOURCED	METHOD OF EXTRACTION
CANDELILLA WAX /EUPHORBIA CERÍFERA		
ALL SKIN TYPES **PARTS USED:** *powder-like waxy substance covering leaves of the plant* **COLOR:** *yellow to tan* **SHELF LIFE:** *3-4 years* **SAFETY CONCERNS:** *none*	*northern Mexican desert and southwestern US*	*leaves and stems are boiled in sulfuric acid*
CARNAUBA WAX /COPERNICIA CERIFERA		
ALL SKIN TYPES **PARTS USED:** *leaves* **COLOR:** *yellow-brown* **SHELF LIFE:** *3-4 years* **SAFETY CONCERNS:** *none*	*Brazil*	*The leaves of the carnauba palm are dried and then beaten to loosen the wax.*

HOW IT IS PROCESSED	HIGHLIGHTED FEATURES	THERAPEUTIC ACTIONS
leaves and stems are first cut and dried and then boiled in sulfuric acid that separates the wax from the plant material	supports skin barrier function	excellent vegan alternative to beeswax, provides gloss and shine, and can give a hard coating (harder than beeswax)
refining and bleaching may occur; check with your supplier	hypoallergenic, emollient	excellent vegan alternative to beeswax, provides gloss and shine, and can give a hard coating (harder than beeswax)

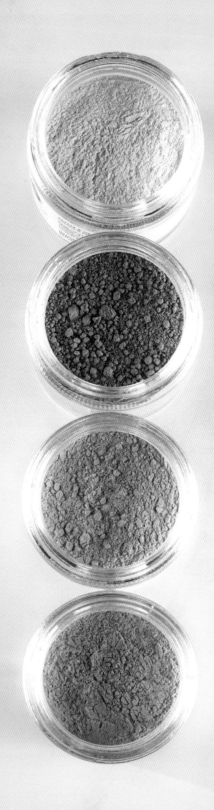

CLAYS

WHAT THEY ARE

Clays are natural minerals from the earth with the power to safely absorb excess oils and toxins from the skin. Depending on where in the world the clay is cultivated, the mineral composition and absorption levels will vary (and, in turn, be appropriate for different skin types).

HOW THEY ARE USED

In beauty formulating, clays are primarily used for facial masks and scrubs, to gently detoxify, exfoliate, clean, and invigorate the skin. Some are also used in soaps as a lathering agent.

Beauty Note!

Here are some of our favorite reasons to use clays:

- They absorb excess oil.
- They bind to toxins and draw them out.
- They clean away dirt.
- They support exfoliation.
- They improve circulation.
- They reduce swelling and inflammation.

CLAYS

	WHERE IT IS SOURCED	METHOD OF EXTRACTION

BENTONITE CLAY /SODIUM BENTONITE

	WHERE IT IS SOURCED	METHOD OF EXTRACTION
CONGESTED/OILY SKIN **COLOR:** cream to gray **SHELF LIFE:** 2–3 years **SAFETY CONCERNS:** none	Clay gathered from its original source deposit. Clay beds that are deposits of weathered volcanic ash, found in the US, specifically Wyoming	Refined and processed in various ways by manufacturers. This can include heating or baking the clay, since the raw clay tends to contain a variety of microorganisms.

FRENCH GREEN CLAY /MONTMORILLONITE (ALSO KNOWN AS ILLITE)

COMBINATION SKIN **COLOR:** light green **SHELF LIFE:** 2–3 years **SAFETY CONCERNS:** none	Clay gathered from its original source deposit. Clay beds that are deposits of decomposed plant materials and iron oxides, which give it its green color, found in France	sun-dried, crushed, and pulverized and dried again

PINK KAOLIN CLAY /ROSE AND WHITE CLAY BLENDED TOGETHER; KAOLINITE AND ILLITE IRON OXIDES

SENSITIVE SKIN **COLOR:** pink **SHELF LIFE:** 2–3 years **SAFETY CONCERNS:** none	Pink kaolin clay is a blend of the white and red kaolin, which is derived from the mined mineral kaolinite found in the southeast regions of the US	refined through a complex process using heat and moisture

ROSE CLAY /KAOLINITE AND ILLITE IRON OXIDES

NORMAL SKIN **COLOR:** rose **SHELF LIFE:** 2–3 years **SAFETY CONCERNS:** none	Rose kaolin clay is a blend of illite and iron oxides with kaolinite, which is derived from the mined mineral kaolinite found in the southeast regions of the US	refined through a complex process using heat and moisture

HIGHLIGHTED FEATURES	THERAPEUTIC ACTIONS
rich in silica, aluminum, and iron, with traces of magnesium, calcium, titanium, and potassium	highly absorbent, detoxifying, effectively pulls oils and toxins from the skin
rich in valuable minerals like magnesium, calcium, potassium, dolomite, silica, manganese, phosphorous, silicon, copper, and selenium	antiseptic, anti-inflammatory, cleansing, detoxifying, highly absorbent, pulls oils and toxins from the skin, stimulates blood flow, and tightens pores
rich in kaolinite silica, iron, magnesium, calcium, sodium, zinc, and minerals	helps stimulate circulation while softly exfoliating and cleansing
rich in kaolinite silica, iron, magnesium, calcium, sodium, zinc, and minerals	anti-inflammatory, removes dead skin cells, tightens pores, fades hyperpigmentation, detoxifying, exfoliant, reduces irritation, increases circulation, regenerates collagen, promotes new cell growth for skin, and regenerates elastin within the skin

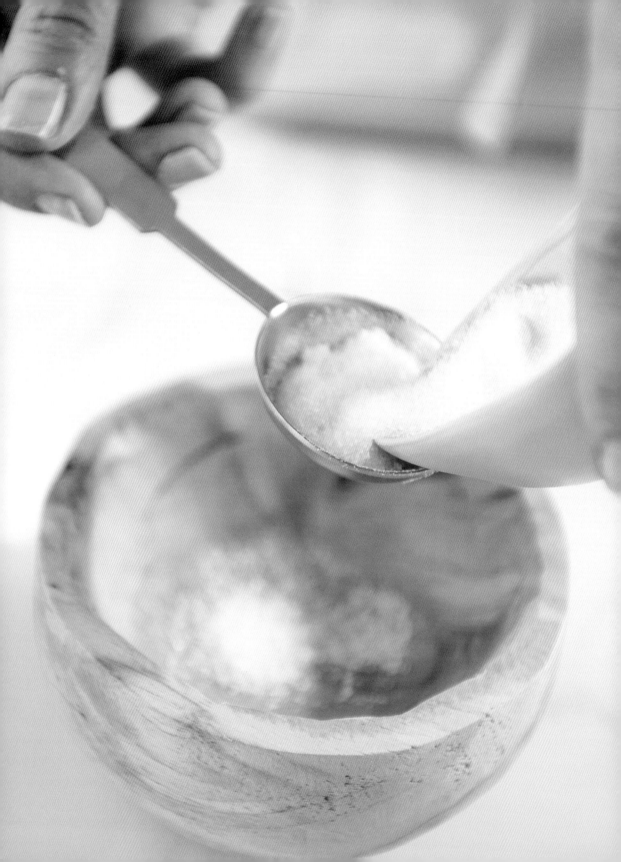

EXFOLIANTS

WHAT THEY ARE

Exfoliants are materials used as ingredients in skincare products to encourage the outermost layer of the skin to slough off dead cells and support healthy skin-cell regeneration from the deeper layers in the epidermis.

Exfoliants include materials like:

— salts: Dead Sea salts, Celtic Sea salts, pink salts, Himalayan salts, Bolivian pink salts, mineral salts, French salts, and Epsom salts

— sugars: organic sugar, brown sugar, and coconut sugar

— flours: grains and powders

— dried plant materials: herbs and spices; finely ground nuts, seeds, and kernels; and even coffee grounds

Beauty Tip!

Use rougher-textured exfoliants for tougher areas on the body like feet, hands, knees, and elbows, and opt for quick-dissolving and softer-feeling powders, flours, grains, herbs, and spices for more sensitive areas like the face. Salts and sugars are extremely stable, while powders, flours, grains, and dried herbs and spices may lose their potency over time.

HOW THEY ARE USED

Exfoliants are used primarily in facial and body scrubs, as well as in cleansers. They can also provide interesting textures to support the look and feel of a product.

We recommend selecting exfoliants that will not be too harsh on the skin, such as finely ground sea salts and organic sugar, since they soften and melt when they come into contact with water. Exfoliants that do not dissolve in water, like finely ground nuts, seeds, kernels, and coffee beans, may cause irritation for those with sensitive and/ or mature skin. In fact, the unevenly ground edges of these particular exfoliant materials may possibly cause tiny microscopic tears on the skin's surface that could weaken the skin's immunity and contribute to signs of premature aging.

	WHERE IT IS SOURCED	METHOD OF EXTRACTION
ALMOND MEAL /PRUNUS DULCIS		
ALL SKIN TYPES **COLOR:** *white* **SHELF LIFE:** *within 6 months* **SAFETY CONCERNS:** *avoid if allergic to tree nuts*	*Origins believed to be from Central Asia*	*harvesting, shelling, and hulling*
DEAD SEA SALTS /MARIS SAL (DEAD SEA SALT)		
ALL SKIN TYPES **COLOR:** *white* **SHELF LIFE:** *indefinite* **SAFETY CONCERNS:** *none*	*Israel, the Dead Sea*	*evaporation ponds*
HEMP SEEDS /CANNABIS SATIVA		
ALL SKIN TYPES **COLOR:** *green and white* **SHELF LIFE:** *within 6 months* **SAFETY CONCERNS:** *none*	*native to Central Asia; now widely cultivated*	*dried seeds collected from harvested and dried flowers*
ORGANIC SUGAR /SUCROSE		
ALL SKIN TYPES **COLOR:** *off-white* **SHELF LIFE:** *indefinite* **SAFETY CONCERNS:** *none*	*grows well in a wide range of climates*	*shredding and squeezing cane stalks*

HOW IT IS PROCESSED	HIGHLIGHTED FEATURES	THERAPEUTIC ACTIONS
After cleaning and sorting nuts are generally left to air dry before being placed into hulling cylinders that crack the shells and vibrating screens that remove the shell. After hulling, the nut is ground into a fine meal.	high in a few key fatty acids, trace amounts of sterols, which can be balancing for the skin	emollient, relieves itchiness and dryness, soothing to symptoms associated with eczema and atopic dermatitis
irrigation canals direct water into shallow evaporation ponds/pools, which then use the sunlight and the dry atmosphere to evaporate the water, leaving behind the salt	mineral-rich and containing high proportions of potassium, magnesium, and bromide	skin soothing, anti-inflammatory, stimulates blood and lymphatic circulation, increased circulation moves trapped fluid from joints, improving joint movement, and reducing stiffness and pain
After cleaning and sorting, seed hull is removed to expose heart of the seed; this can be done using large machinery that vibrates, using water and air pressure, or by hand.	rich in vitamin E, essential fatty acids, and protein	anti-inflammatory, cell regenerative
cane juice is boiled down and centrifuged to separate the molasses, and then evaporated to create the crystals	natural humectants; brings moisture to the skin and balances pH of skin	soothing, balancing, evening out tone, supports skin microbiome

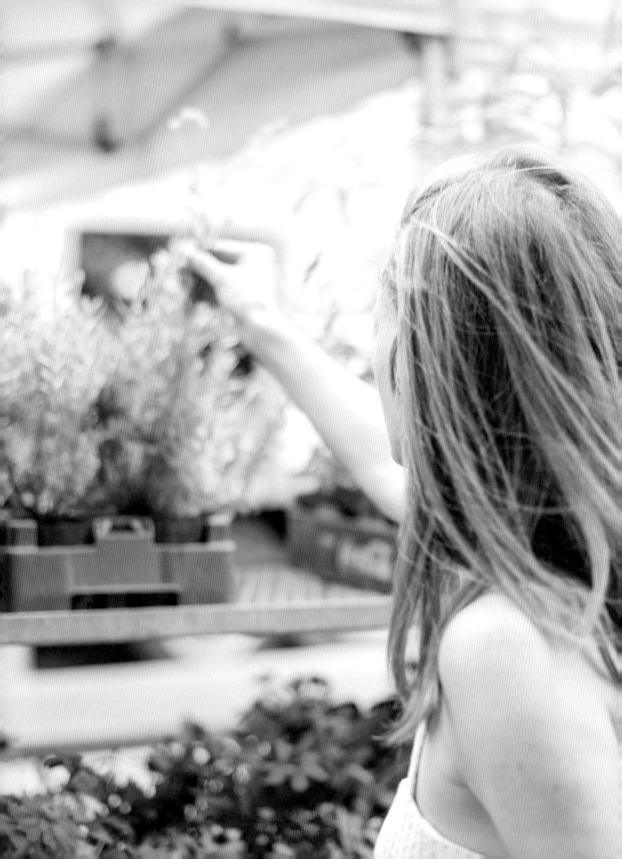

HERBS AND SPICES

WHAT THEY ARE

Herbs and spices contribute many effective components to botanical skin-care recipes. From a culinary perspective, the term *herbs* generally refers to the leaves of the plant, while *spices* refers to all the other plant parts, like roots, seeds, bark, flowers, and fruit. Plant medicine practitioners (herbalists), however, don't necessarily differentiate between the two and find therapeutic uses in all parts of the plants.

Beauty Tip!

If you decide to use fresh herbs and spices in your recipes, make sure you use the product immediately after blending, to prevent it from spoiling. For example, our Quick and Fresh Cucumber-Thyme Body Scrub (see page 214) includes fresh cucumber, thyme, and tarragon, so it doesn't keep well and should be used within minutes of blending.

HOW THEY ARE USED

You will find herbs and spices in many of our beauty recipes: oils, cleansers, masks, scrubs, and gels. They can make up the bulk of a plant-based beauty recipe and offer a wide range of dynamic healing properties.

In our recipes, we use both fresh and dried herbs and spices, and we select them specifically with their therapeutic properties in mind. In some recipes, such as cleansers, scrubs, or masks, we use these materials directly, while in other recipes we use their infusions or extracts. Either way, we incorporate their therapeutic components into the recipe to support and enhance the effectiveness of the product.

For example, we may choose to use dried and ground calendula flowers in a facial mask to reduce inflammation and soothe irritation, while we may decide to use calendula-infused olive oil in a recipe for a facial serum for the same purpose: reducing inflammation and soothing irritation.

Herbs and spices can add great dimension to a recipe's aroma and texture, as well as offer nutrients, minerals, and healing properties.

HERBS AND SPICES

	WHERE IT IS SOURCED	METHOD OF EXTRACTION

CALENDULA /CALENDULA OFFICINALIS

ALL SKIN TYPES PARTS USED: *flowers* COLOR: *light yellow* SHELF LIFE: *2 years* SAFETY CONCERNS: *none*	*grows well in warm, temperate climates*	*fresh flowers are picked and air dried on screens*

CHAMOMILE, GERMAN /MATRICARIA RECUTITA

ALL SKIN TYPES PARTS USED: *flowers* COLOR: *pale yellow* SHELF LIFE: *2 years* SAFETY CONCERNS: *none*	*native to Eastern Europe; now grows abundantly in the US*	*fresh flowers are picked and air dried on screens*

COMFREY /SYMPHYTUM OFFICINALE

ALL SKIN TYPES PARTS USED: *leaves* COLOR: *green* SHELF LIFE: *2 years* SAFETY CONCERNS: *avoid using on open wounds*	*hardy plant that is an annual and is able to grow anywhere; native to Europe*	*fresh leaves are harvested and air-dried on screens*

FENNEL /FOENICULUM VULGARE

ALL SKIN TYPES PARTS USED: *seeds* COLOR: *gray* SHELF LIFE: *2 years* SAFETY CONCERNS: *avoid during first trimester of pregnancy or while undergoing any estrogenic cancer treatment*	*hardy in mild climates and some cold climates, drought tolerant, able to grow in a variety of locations, native to southern Europe*	*flowers are collected as seeds become visible and dried until seeds shake away*

GINGER /ZINGZIBER OFFICINALE

ALL SKIN TYPES PARTS USED: *roots* COLOR: *light gold* SHELF LIFE: *2 years* SAFETY CONCERNS: *none*	*native to East Asia, now grown in warm subtropical areas*	*fresh roots are harvested and smaller root shoots are scraped away; roots are chopped into small pieces and dried on screens or dehydrated*

HOW IT IS PROCESSED	HIGHLIGHTED FEATURES	THERAPEUTIC ACTIONS
dried flowers are finely ground into a powder	rich in flavonoids	anti-inflammatory, antibacterial, wound healing, skin soothing
dried flowers are finely ground into a powder	highly anti-inflammatory	anti-inflammatory, wound healing, antibacterial, soothing, calming
dried leaves are finely ground into a powder	rich in allantoin	wound healing, muscle relaxing, anti-inflammatory, antibacterial, astringent
dried seeds are finely ground into a powder	rich in amino acids that strengthen blood and soothe digestive problems	anti-inflammatory, antibacterial, wound healing, skin soothing
dried roots are chopped and finely ground into a powder	rich in antimicrobials and supports circulation	warming, cleansing, detoxifying, energizing, improves circulation, brightening

	WHERE IT IS SOURCED	METHOD OF EXTRACTION
LAVENDER /LAVANDULA ANGUSTIFOLIA		
ALL SKIN TYPES **PARTS USED:** *flowers* **COLOR:** *pale lavender* **SHELF LIFE:** *2 years* **SAFETY CONCERNS:** *none*	*native to the south of France; now grows in a variety of areas that can withstand heat and drought; some of our favorites are from Oregon, Canada, India, and the UK*	*fresh flower clusters are picked and air-dried on screens*
MATCHA /CAMELLIA SINENSIS		
ALL SKIN TYPES **PARTS USED:** *leaves* **COLOR:** *bright green* **SHELF LIFE:** *1 year (keep cool or refrigerated)* **SAFETY CONCERNS:** *none*	*Japan*	*Processing matcha has many steps: First the plant must be shaded for about 3 weeks before the new tender leaves can be picked, then once picked they are lightly steamed, and then sent through an air-drying machine, and the veins of the leaves are separated out. What remains then is ground into match powder.*
MUSTARD /BRASSICA ALBA OR BRASSICA JUNCEA		
ALL SKIN TYPES **PARTS USED:** *seeds* **COLOR:** *yellow or brown* **SHELF LIFE:** *2 years* **SAFETY CONCERNS:** *none*	*native to the Himalayas; now grows in the US, the UK, Canada, and Denmark*	*flowers are collected as seeds become visible and dried until the seeds shake away*
TURMERIC /CURCUMA LONGA		
ALL SKIN TYPES **PARTS USED:** *roots* **COLOR:** *bright orange* **SHELF LIFE:** *2 years* **SAFETY CONCERNS:** *none*	*native to East Asia; now grown in warm subtropical areas*	*fresh roots are harvested and smaller root shoots are scraped away; roots are chopped into small pieces and dried on screens or dehydrated*

HOW IT IS PROCESSED	HIGHLIGHTED FEATURES	THERAPEUTIC ACTIONS
dried flowers are finely ground into a powder	anti-inflammatory and wound healing	anti-inflammatory, skin soothing, antibacterial, antiseptic, sedative
dried and ground	contains chlorophyll, antioxidants that combat free radical damage and oxidative stress to the skin, anti-inflammatory, cell regenerative	antioxidant, rejuvenating, brightening, energizing, balancing to skin's own oil content, detoxifying, cleansing, excellent for sensitive and mature skin
dried seeds are finely ground into a powder	rich in antioxidants, brightening, boosts circulation, warming	wound healing, anti-inflammatory, cleansing, pain relieving, yellow mustard powders are more heating
dried roots are chopped and finely ground into a powder	rich in curcumin, an antioxidant; anti-inflammatory and regenerative	anti-inflammatory, antioxidant, antibacterial, wound healing, balances oils in skin, brightening, evens out skin tone

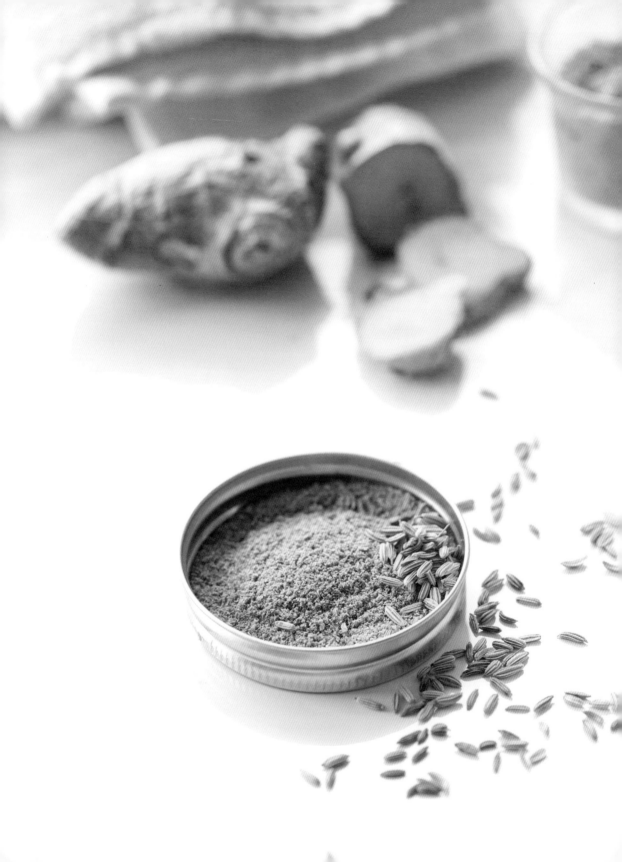

FLOURS AND GRAINS

WHAT THEY ARE

Flours are grains that have been dried and ground into powder. For our purposes, flours also include oats, rice, and their respective brans, as well as dried legumes, like chickpeas or lentils. These ingredients provide a spectrum of lovely properties that contribute to both the therapeutic actions and the touch and feel of the product.

HOW THEY ARE USED

Flours are best used in facial and body scrubs, cleansers, and masks. They are easy to work with and have a soft feel on the skin. You can grind your own oats into powder and then add it to a facial mask or cleanser to help balance out uneven skin tone and soothe irritation. Or you can add rice bran flour to boost the delivery of some essential fatty acids directly to the skin.

Beauty Tip!

Keep your flours away from direct sunlight and any moisture, since they can easily become compromised and go rancid.

FLOURS AND GRAINS

	WHERE IT IS SOURCED	METHOD OF EXTRACTION

CHICKPEA FLOUR /CICER ARIETINUM

ALL SKIN TYPES **PARTS USED:** *legumes* **COLOR:** *light yellow* **SHELF LIFE:** *1 year* **SAFETY CONCERNS:** *none*	*temperate climates, but grows best when avoiding frost*	*mature beans are collected from pods*

OAT FLOUR /AVENA SATIVA

ALL SKIN TYPES **PARTS USED:** *seeds* **COLOR:** *white to gray* **SHELF LIFE:** *1 year* **SAFETY CONCERNS:** *none*	*temperate climates; low heat requirements and can tolerate rain*	*seeds are collected from dried grasses*

RICE BRAN POWDER /ORYZA SATIVA

ALL SKIN TYPES **PARTS USED:** *seeds* **COLOR:** *tan* **SHELF LIFE:** *1 year* **SAFETY CONCERNS:** *none*	*wet climates*	*seeds are collected from dried grasses*

TAPIOCA STARCH /MANIHOT ESCULENTA

ALL SKIN TYPES **PARTS USED:** *roots* **COLOR:** *white* **SHELF LIFE:** *1 year* **SAFETY CONCERNS:** *cassava should not be eaten raw or unpeeled (poisonous)*	*tropical and subtropical regions*	*roots are pulled and carefully stored*

HOW IT IS PROCESSED	HIGHLIGHTED FEATURES	THERAPEUTIC ACTIONS
a centrifuge cylinder removes the legume coating, and then they are finely ground	draws out impurities, zinc improves immunity of skin	lightening and brightening skin, evening out skin tone, antibacterial, anti-acne, wound healing
includes threshing (hitting the seeds out of the grass) and winnowing (loosening and blowing away the feathery covering); and then dried oats are ground into a fine flour	unique antioxidants work as effective anti-irritants	anti-inflammatory, cleansing, exfoliant, wound healing, moisturizing, antioxidant
the bran, the outer coating of the seed, is removed through vibration and centrifuge and then finely ground	high in antioxidants and sterols that protect the skin and encourage cell regenerative actions	anti-aging, antioxidant, moisturizing, reparative, high in EFA
roots are peeled, soaked, and mashed, and then all the liquid is squeezed out, leaving behind a pulp that is then dried and ground into a flour.	high in calcium and carbohydrates	skin soothing and softening, immune protective for acid mantle of skin

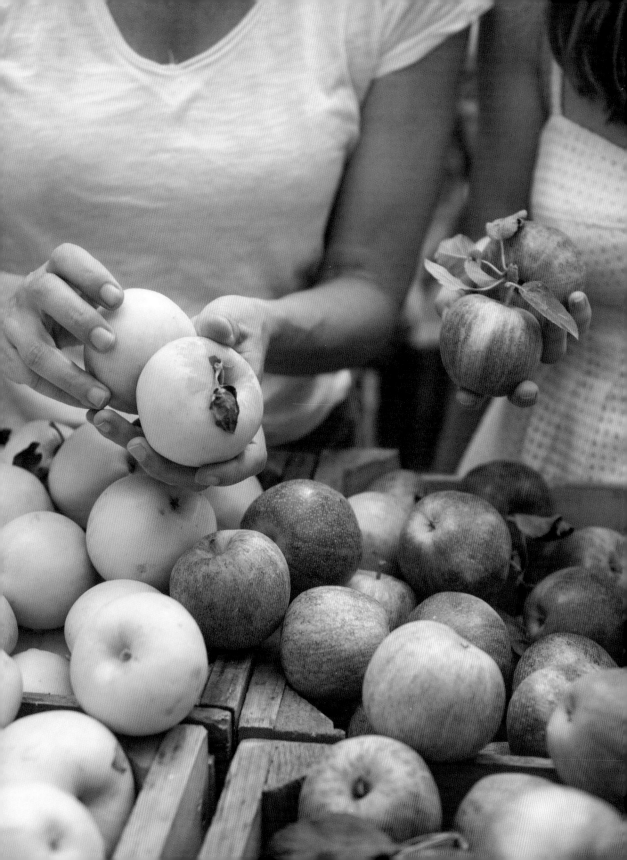

FRUITS AND VEGETABLES

WHAT THEY ARE

Fresh fruits and vegetables offer powerful results when used as ingredients in freshly prepared skincare recipes. Many of their components, like vitamins, nutrients, minerals, and enzymes, can feed the skin in many of the same ways that they nourish and strengthen our bodies. When fruits and vegetables are prepared correctly, which usually entails blending, grinding, and/or mashing, the skin can more easily absorb what it needs.

HOW THEY ARE USED

Fresh fruits and vegetables are best used in masks and scrubs. For example, blended berries can give an immediate boost to dull, tired skin, while freshly ground greens and herbs can infuse the cells of the skin with much-needed minerals and nutrients. You'll find some specific fruits and vegetables mentioned in our recipes, but we also suggest you experiment with items you can find fresh at your local market—you can research their nutrition content and see how they might be used for skin health and healing.

Beauty Tip!

The trick is using these fresh ingredients as soon as they are prepared— their freshness won't stay and the potency of the desired enzymes and nutrients will diminish quickly.

	WHERE IT IS SOURCED	METHOD OF EXTRACTION

APPLE /MALUS DOMESTICA

ALL SKIN TYPES **COLOR:** *pale beige* **SHELF LIFE:** *1 year* **SAFETY CONCERNS:** *none*	*North America, Europe, Asia, and Africa*	*picking fresh fruit*

BLUEBERRY /VACCINIUM CYANOCOCCUS

ALL SKIN TYPES **COLOR:** *deep indigo blue* **SHELF LIFE:** *1 year* **SAFETY CONCERNS:** *none*	*North America, Europe, Asia, and Africa*	*picking fresh berries*

CARROT /DAUCUS CAROTA

ALL SKIN TYPES **COLOR:** *bright orange* **SHELF LIFE:** *1 year* **SAFETY CONCERNS:** *none*	*hardy, grows in a variety of locations*	*harvesting fresh roots*

STRAWBERRY /FRAGARIA × ANANASSA

ALL SKIN TYPES **COLOR:** *pink* **SHELF LIFE:** *1 year* **SAFETY CONCERNS:** *none*	*North America, Europe, Asia, and Africa*	*picking fresh berries*

RASPBERRY /RUBUS IDAEUS

ALL SKIN TYPES **COLOR:** *magenta to deep red* **SHELF LIFE:** *1 year* **SAFETY CONCERNS:** *none*	*North America, Europe, Asia, and Africa*	*picking fresh berries*

WHEAT GRASS /TRITICUM AESTIVUM

ALL SKIN TYPES **COLOR:** *bright green* **SHELF LIFE:** *1 year* **SAFETY CONCERNS:** *none*	*can grow anywhere in a greenhouse and indoors*	*harvesting fresh young grass*

HOW IT IS PROCESSED	HIGHLIGHTED FEATURES	THERAPEUTIC ACTIONS
Clean, sort, peel, and slice. Dry in a dehydrator and then grind into a fine powder.	rich in pectins	exfoliant, clears pores, soothes inflammation, healing, rich in vitamins, supports elasticin, cell regeneration
Clean, sort, and then quickly blanch to "pop" the skin. Dry in a dehydrator and then grind into a fine powder.	rich in flavonoids and antioxidants, particularly anthocyanin	antioxidant, anti-aging, rich in vitamin C, supports healing and collagen, anti-inflammatory, balancing
Clean, sort, peel, and slice. Dry in a dehydrator, and then grind into a fine powder.	antioxidants, beta-carotene, vitamin C	cell regenerative, anti-inflammatory, cleansing, detoxifying, anti-aging, rich in vitamins and minerals
Dry in a dehydrator, and then grind into a fine powder.	rich in salicylic acid	brightening, lightening, evens out skin tone, exfoliating, improves circulation, antioxidant, antibacterial
Clean, sort. Dry in a dehydrator, and then grind into a fine powder.	rich in antioxidants and ellagic acid	anti-aging, evens out skin tone, antioxidant, rich in vitamin C, anti-inflammatory, immune boosting
Tender shoots are first juiced. Juice is then evaporated, and dried plant material or pulp is left over and further dehydrated and powdered.	rich in amino acids, vitamins, and enzymes	cell regenerative, anti-inflammatory, cleansing, detoxifying, anti-aging, rich in vitamins and minerals

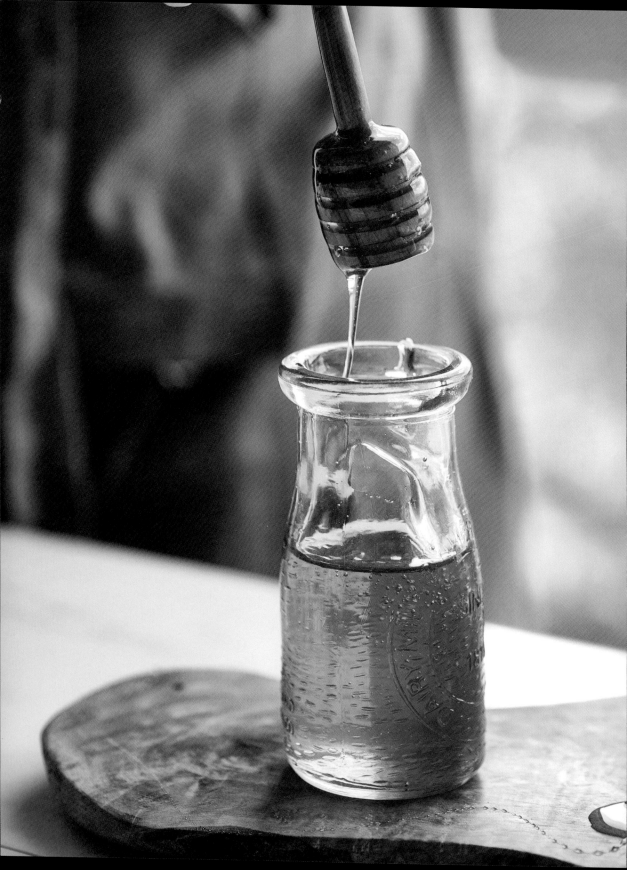

OTHER INGREDIENTS

WHAT THEY ARE

This category includes ingredients that cannot necessarily be grouped together on their own or that do not fit into another class. But their role in the recipe provides a very specific function, through both their relation to the other ingredients and their therapeutic function. They include vegetable glycerin, honey, aloe vera juice/gel, and surfactants, such as castile soap, gums, and antioxidants.

HOW THEY ARE USED

The functions of these other ingredients include attracting moisture to the skin, preventing rancidity, supporting emulsification, lathering, and contributing to the product's texture. You can find them in our recipes for cleansers, gels, oils, and scrubs, and in most instances they are used not in large percentages but rather as supporting components to enhance the formula's therapeutic effects, longevity, and feel.

Beauty Tip!

Working with some of these ingredients may take a little practice, since they can sometimes be sticky and challenging to mix with other recipe components. We have offered a few procedural suggestions. For example, in our Almond Milk Facial Cleanser recipe (see page 156), we instruct you to mix the xanthan gum into the vegetable glycerin before incorporating the castile soap and the almond milk; by following this procedure exactly, you will avoid having your cleanser separate and you will create a consistency that feels silky on the skin.

	WHERE IT IS SOURCED	METHOD OF EXTRACTION
ALOE VERA /ALOE BARBADENSIS		
ALL SKIN TYPES **PARTS USED:** *center inner section of leaves* **COLOR:** *clear to pale yellow* **VISCOSITY:** *slightly heavier than milk-like (juice); thick and gel-like (gel)* **SHELF LIFE:** *up to 10 days (refrigerate immediately after opening)* **SAFETY CONCERNS:** *none*	*Rio Grande Valley, Texas, and Mexico*	*cutting and scraping gel from inner leaf; use of a separator*
CASTILE SOAP		
OILY/COMBINATION SKIN **PARTS USED:** *n/a* **COLOR:** *clear to pale yellow* **VISCOSITY:** *water-like to milk-like* **SHELF LIFE:** *2–3 years* **SAFETY CONCERNS:** *do not ingest*	*originated from Castile, Spain; now readily available anywhere soap is manufactured*	*process of saponification*
HONEY		
ALL SKIN TYPES **PARTS USED:** *by-product of bee nectar collection* **COLOR:** *golden* **VISCOSITY:** *thick and gooey* **SHELF LIFE:** *2–3 years* **SAFETY CONCERNS:** *none*	*worldwide*	*gathered by beekeepers*
ORGANIC HIGH PROOF ALCOHOL /ETHANOL		
ALL SKIN TYPES **PARTS USED:** *n/a* **COLOR:** *clear* **VISCOSITY:** *water-like* **SHELF LIFE:** *indefinite* **SAFETY CONCERNS:** *do not ingest*	*worldwide*	*distillation*

HOW IT IS PROCESSED	HIGHLIGHTED FEATURES	THERAPEUTIC ACTIONS
washed, cut, drained, filtered, homogenized, pasteurized, and stabilized	skin penetrator	antiseptic, anti-inflammatory, wound healing, soothes sun damage, moisturizing
adding either sodium hydroxide or potassium hydroxide to vegetable oils	surfactant	lifts and rinses dirt away from skin, offers a foaming action to product
honey extractor	filtering	antibacterial, antioxidant, improves circulation
cleaning, sorting grapes, mashing, and soaking	as a menstruum, solubilizer	used as a vehicle to absorb chemical constituents from plant materials and to solubilize essential oils into water

	WHERE IT IS SOURCED	METHOD OF EXTRACTION
VEGETABLE GLYCERIN /GLYCERIN		
ALL SKIN TYPES PARTS USED: *by-product of saponified vegetable oil* COLOR: *clear* VISCOSITY: *very thick and viscous* SHELF LIFE: *2–3 years* SAFETY CONCERNS: *none*	*worldwide*	*multistep process, involves saponification and distillation*
VITAMIN E /TOCOPHEROL		
ALL SKIN TYPES PARTS USED: *isolated tocopherols from vegetable oils* COLOR: *yellow to orange* VISCOSITY: *thick and gooey* SHELF LIFE: *2–3 years* SAFETY CONCERNS: *none*	*found anywhere nut and seed oils high in tocopherols are processed, though China is a large supplier*	*chemical process to isolate tocopherols*
WITCH HAZEL EXTRACT /HAMAMELIS VIRGINIANA		
OILY/COMBINATION SKIN PARTS USED: *leaves and bark* COLOR: *clear* VISCOSITY: *water-like* SHELF LIFE: *1–2 years* SAFETY CONCERNS: *none*	*northeastern regions of the US*	*extract in water and alcohol or hydrosol*
XANTHUM GUM		
ALL SKIN TYPES PARTS USED: *n/a* COLOR: *white* VISCOSITY: *n/a* SHELF LIFE: *indefinite* SAFETY CONCERNS: *none*	*originally discovered in a lab of the USDA in the 1960s*	*microbial fermentation of the microorganism Xanthonmonas campestris using different sugars*

HOW IT IS PROCESSED	HIGHLIGHTED FEATURES	THERAPEUTIC ACTIONS
refining glycerin involves balancing its pH, heating, and using activated charcoal to remove color	humectant	attract water to the skin, and keep water in the skin
the isolated tocopherols are often added to soybean oil, so make sure the soy oil is GMO-free	used to stabilize formulations	antioxidant, prevents rancidity of butters and vegetable oils
leaves and branches are washed and made into pulp, soaked, and distilled or made into a tincture	astringent, antiseptic	astringent, antiseptic, wound healing, anti-inflammatory, antibacterial
fermentation and then drying and powdering	thickener, forms gels, helps emulsify oil and water	adds texture and softness to a formula; should be used at a small percentage and best to mix with glycerin first

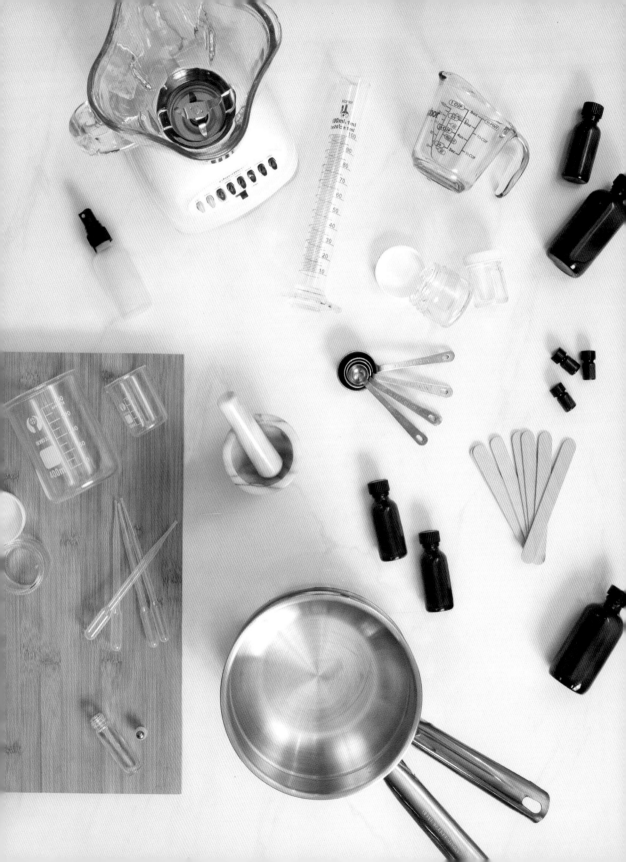

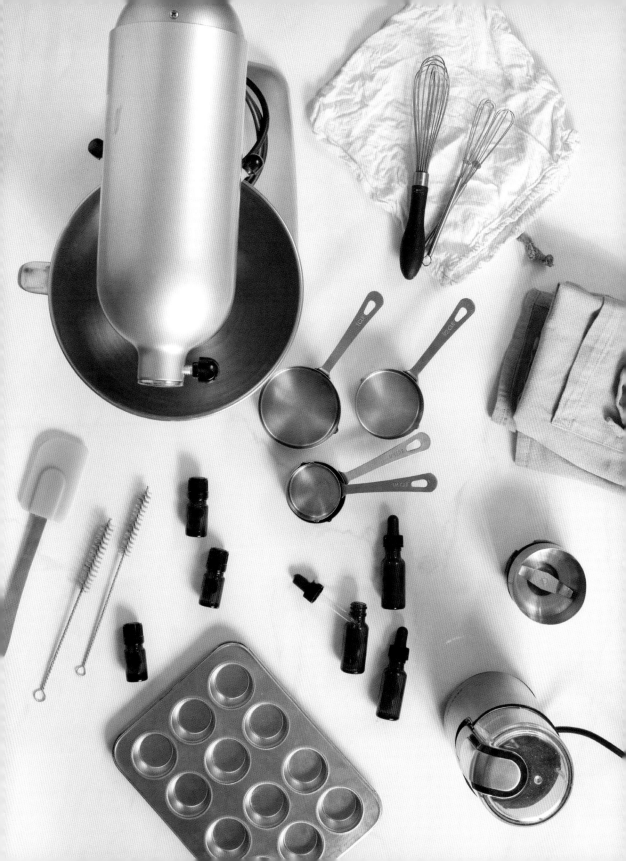

WHAT YOU NEED IN YOUR BEAUTY FORMULATION KITCHEN

Setting yourself up with the right tools is step one in do-it-yourself beauty formulating. Whether you plan to make products for yourself or loved ones or you venture into developing your own beauty line, your kitchen items will be central to your success. We recommend that you purchase dedicated equipment for your product blending so you can control what ingredients touch your tools and easily keep everything sterilized.

Your beauty kitchen **must-haves**:

✓ **Stainless-steel double boiler:** You can select a 1-quart or 2-quart size. This item will allow you to melt butters and waxes at low temperatures and incorporate nut and seed oils without worrying that the heat will affect their chemical components.

✓ **Stainless-steel measuring cups and spoons:** The spoons should start at ¼ teaspoon and go up to 1 tablespoon; the cups should start at ¼ cup and go up to 1 cup. Stainless steel makes for easy cleanup and sterilizing.

✓ **Glass measuring pitchers:** You will need at least two 1-cup sizes and one 2-cup size. Glass measuring pitchers are great for pouring heated preparations and gently warming up butters and waxes that have started to solidify. They also clean up well and are easy to sterilize.

✓ **Blender:** This is an especially important machine if you love making cream and want to hone your emulsifying skills. A blender that holds 5 or 6 cups should do the trick. Make sure the pitcher is glass, the blades are stainless steel, and the unit can be taken apart for no-hassle cleaning.

✓ **Mixer:** You can opt for either a handheld mixer or a stand mixer. Be sure the blades are stainless steel and removable, and check to be sure you have a nice selection of speeds. Opt for a mixing bowl that is either stainless steel or glass.

✓ **Plastic pipettes:** These disposable measuring devices are very useful when incorporating essential oils into your products. Pipettes help you measure out drops and avoid contamination or accidental intermixing with other essential oils. We generally use pipettes ranging in size from 5 ml to 7 ml.

✓ **Small glass dropper bottles:** These small, colored (amber, blue, green, etc.— just never clear) glass bottles are typically 5 ml to 10 ml in size, with a plastic orifice reducer on the top, and are used to mix your essential oils synergy before the oil blend is incorporated into a product.

✓ **Glass bottles and jars:** Once you have made your product, you will need to transfer it to an appropriate bottle or jar. It is always a good idea to have a selection of glass bottles (both colored and clear) and jars on hand. The decision between colored glass and clear glass depends on a few different considerations:

1. Generally, it is the best practice to store all essential oils and fixed oils (carrier oils) in dark glass to help maintain their stability and shelf life, since the dark glass reduces the harm light may have on the molecules of the oils.

2. Clear glass bottles are nice to use for products when you want to show off how pretty they look. And we often prefer to store our hydrosols in clear glass because that way we can monitor their freshness and stability more easily.

There are many different sizes, colors, and tops available, so the choice really depends on your preference. Here's our quick list of tops and bottle sizes you might consider having on hand:

- *flip-tops*
- *glass droppers with rubber screw tops*
- *twist tops*
- *spray tops*
- *foaming tops*
- *treatment pump*
- *jars: 1-, 2-, and 4-ounce jars with twist tops*
- *bottles: 1- and 2-ounce bottles. The tops are usually interchangeable, so if you purchase bottles with dropper lids, you can often swap them for others, such as twist tops or spray tops.*

There are also container options for specialized products:

- *roll-ons: usually come in a 0.33-ounce glass tube with a small rolling ball*
- *inhalers: stainless-steel and plastic (most common) containers*
- *lip balm: containers typically range from 0.15 ounce to 0.25 ounce; standard plastic lip balm tubes are 0.15 ounce in size.*

- ✓ **Plastic bottles:** Although we are not big advocates of using plastic containers, especially since there is growing evidence of their negative effects not only on our health but also on the health and safety of the environment,[1] we occasionally find ourselves in situations where using plastic is the best choice, for ease of transport or weight reasons. For example, we use a 1-ounce plastic bottle with a flip-top for our hand sanitizer. That way it is light when we are lugging it around. Plastic is also a smart pick if your product needs to be squeezed out a bit.

  In these instances we strongly advise you to make sure any plastic container you use is BPA-free (meaning free from the chemical compound bisphenol A, which has been linked to cancer and hormone imbalances)[2] and to find plastic that is made of polyethylene terephthalate (PET). PET plastic should be clearly stamped on the bottom and is available in clear and dark colors.

  One final thought on plastic containers—never allow your essential oils to make direct contact with them because the oils will eat through the plastic.

- ✓ **Labels:** It is important to keep track of a product's ingredients and the date you made the product, so we suggest labeling all your jars and bottles. A simple white matte address label will do the trick. Or you can get creative and design something gorgeous.

- ✓ **Mixing tools (disposable wooden mixing sticks or metal or glass rods):** Disposable wooden sticks are great if you want to use a clean implement every time you combine ingredients or test a new product. We have found them at beauty supply stores, since they are often used for waxing. Popsicle sticks also work quite well. But the glass and metal rods are actually the best because you can easily sanitize them after every use. Keep in mind that any kitchen utensil that has been previously used for food or other purposes has the potential for carrying remnants. Therefore, we suggest you either keep a nice supply of disposable wooden mixing sticks handy or collect a few metal or glass mixing rods.

✓ **Apron:** We think everyone should wear an apron when they formulate because things can, and often do, get messy.

✓ **Whisk:** This blending tool will really help achieve that luscious consistency we are so often seeking, especially in our creams. It is also useful for fully incorporating ingredients when blending certain gels. Try to find a baby size (with the whisk part about 5 inches long) and one the next size up. You can often find these at kitchen supply shops.

✓ **Spatula:** We don't want you to waste one drop of your waxes, butters, or oils, so be sure to have a spatula on hand to easily scrape your mixing bowls and make use of every last bit. A silicone-topped one is best.

✓ **Alcohol:** No, not the kind required for cocktails! We mean good old-fashioned rubbing alcohol (also known as isopropyl alcohol). This is one of the best solvents, and it cuts through grease and eliminates greasy residue in an impressive way. So after you wash your equipment with soap and hot water and dry it off, we advise a wipe-down with alcohol to ensure everything is super-sanitized. This same approach should extend to your product containers before filling them up.

✓ **Cutting board:** Whether you are preparing dried plant material for an herbal infusion or dicing up fruit for a facial mask, we recommend having cutting boards around. They will protect your other surfaces and knives and give you a dedicated space for chopping plant material. We gravitate toward natural wood or bamboo surfaces, but the choice is yours.

✓ **Mason jars:** These iconic jars with airtight twist tops come in a wide range of sizes and are useful for almost everything we do. You can use them to make herbal infusions, to store creams and body butters, and so much more. The possibilities are endless.

Nice-to-haves for your beauty kitchen:

✓ **Glass beakers:** These clear measuring containers are a treasure when you wish to precisely blend formulations and then pour them right into product bottles (especially those with small openings). Beakers usually come with a pourable lip and in sizes as small as 10 ml.

✓ **Spice grinder:** When you feel ready to start making your very own dried fruit facial scrubs, a spice grinder will be your best friend. Keep in mind that spice grinders are also sold as coffee bean grinders and that a small size will suffice.

✓ **Dehydrator:** There is really nothing like dehydrating your own fruit and veggies for homemade scrubs. We noticed that the colors and quality are superior to store-bought dried varieties. So, when you are ready to step up your beauty blending game, a dehydrator should be on the top of your list.

✓ **Mortar and pestle:** These tools have been used for thousands of years to prepare plant ingredients by crushing and grinding them into a powder or paste. It is helpful to have a mortar and pestle for making powdered ingredients from scratch, as long as you have the arm muscle and some patience. Plus, they provide a nice decorative touch. They come in stone, marble, and other hard materials.

Psst! ⌒○

Dehydrators are pricey and also require adequate space for storage and use, so plan accordingly.

✓ **Silicone baking trays:** These flexible and colorful baking trays can be found in cooking supply stores or online and are a smart choice for making lotion bars. The nonstick silicone material helps ensure easy removal, and the selection of fun shapes and sizes means you can get really creative.

✓ **Bottle brushes:** Cleaning kitchen tools and bottles can be tricky, especially those hard-to-reach areas. With bottle brushes on hand, you will have a cleaning companion to help get into those tight spots your fingers can't reach. Using bottle brushes is also a sustainable practice—the more bottles you can thoroughly clean and reuse, the better.

✓ **Hemp cloth:** If you decide to make almond milk—a starring ingredient in our amazing Almond Milk Facial Cleanser (see page 156)—from scratch, you will need to have a hemp cloth on hand. Hemp cloth is inexpensive and can last for years if you properly wash, dry, and store it after each use.

Psst! 🗨

Don't get hemp cloth confused with cheesecloth—the results will be dramatically different.

Tips for Keeping a Microbe-Free Kitchen

As botanical beauty formulators, we feel passionately that the products we make should not be wholly dependent on preservatives to stay microbe-free. We embrace the motto that "less is more" and prefer to emphasize whole-plant-based ingredients and their amazing and complex therapeutic properties and how they naturally contribute to the product's efficacy and stability.

In light of this, we have decided not to include any preservatives, naturally derived or synthetic, in our recipes. Instead, we want to share a few of our kitchen-conscious tips, so that your recipes stay fresh and avoid contamination.

1. KEEP YOUR KITCHEN AND EQUIPMENT CLEAN AND STERILE.

— Thoroughly wash and sanitize pots, blenders, mixers, spatulas, spoons, measuring cups and spoons, bowls, and the jars your finished products will be poured into. Put your dishwasher on the hottest setting and wipe down all kitchen tools with rubbing alcohol.

— Wear vinyl or latex examination gloves and change them as needed if you touch something that hasn't been cleaned.

— Make sure all tools are perfectly dry before use.

— Avoid plastic kitchen tools, since they are more challenging to sanitize.

— Wipe down countertops and surface areas of your workspace with 70 to 90 percent rubbing alcohol, which is easily found in many drugstores.

2. STORE YOUR RAW MATERIALS PROPERLY. INSPECT THEM CAREFULLY BEFORE USE.

— Keep track of expiration dates on all your ingredients.

— Make sure ingredients are stored properly (refrigerate them, use glass containers, always keep them away from heat, tightly cap bottles, etc.) and have not "turned."

— Keep a well-organized recipe book and take notes on how the ingredients looked, smelled, and felt when you removed them from their containers.

3. CHOOSE INGREDIENTS THAT ARE ALREADY SELF-PRESERVING.

— Refer to our ingredient charts (beginning on page 68) and look at shelf-life guidelines. Purchase smaller amounts of ingredients that spoil more quickly and larger quantities of ingredients that are more stable.

— Avoid including water in recipes when possible. And if you do use water, make sure it is distilled and not tap or spring. Distilled water is water that has had most of its impurities removed through the process of distillation. And water that has had most of its impurities removed usually becomes contaminated with bacteria, yeast, and mold *less rapidly* than purified or tap water does. But always be aware that any product that includes water, distilled or otherwise, and does not contain a preservative will eventually go bad.

4. CHOOSE PACKAGING THAT REDUCES CHANCES OF CONTAMINATION.

— Use glass containers as much as possible, since they can be easily sterilized and will help keep the product stable.

— Make sure lids and caps are affixed tightly and air space in the container is minimal.

5. USE YOUR PRODUCTS MINDFULLY.

— If you want the recipe to last more than a couple of days, avoid sticking your hands and fingers into the jar or bottle. Instead, dispense the product with a clean spoon, wooden stick, or disposable utensil.

— Keep the cap or lid on the container when a product is not in use.

— Avoid getting water into the product.

— Store the product at a constant temperature—don't take it in and out of the fridge or leave it in a parked car on a hot day.

6. ADD ANTIOXIDANTS.

— An antioxidant is not a preservative.[3] People often confuse the two. Explained simply, a preservative prevents the growth of bacteria, mold, and yeast, whereas an antioxidant prevents the process of oxidation, which accelerates the ingredient's natural process of degradation. A preservative prevents harmful microbes from contaminating the product, whereas an antioxidant keeps the product stable and from going rancid.

We can often tell when a vegetable oil goes "rancid" because the odor and color change. Antioxidants can help lengthen the shelf life of carrier oils, butters, and waxes and may be added directly to the fixed oil or incorporated during your formulating. Examples of antioxidants include:

- **Vitamin E (tocopherol):** An antioxidant extracted and isolated from fixed oils that have high percentages of natural antioxidants. It is most often extracted and isolated from soy, corn, or sugar beets. These crops, if not certified USDA organic, are most likely genetically modified, so it is best to ask your supplier about the source.

- **Rosemary extract:** An antioxidant extracted from rosemary leaves using the CO_2 supercritical extraction method. It is a thick, viscous material rich with the herb's complex array of essential oils and antimicrobial phytochemicals. We have found that the $CO2$ extract of rosemary is an effective stabilizer and prevents rapid deterioration.

- **Grapefruit seed extract:** An extract of the grapefruit seed that exhibits antifungal and antioxidant properties. It's not our favorite antioxidant because there has been evidence that in some brands the carrier in which it is diluted is composed primarily of synthetic compounds; however, there are many who swear by its effectiveness. Our advice would be to contact your supplier to make certain that its components have no concerning synthetic residues.

Measurements: When to Use Volume, When to Use Weight, and Why Your 1-Ounce Bottle May Not Fill to the Brim

You may notice that we provide measurements in volume, like teaspoons and tablespoons, in our recipes. We have done this to simplify the process of "cooking up kitchen beauty," so you can use tools that are readily available and easily found in an already existing kitchen.

Please note that serious beauty product formulators, who scale up the quantities produced and want to ensure recipes stay consistent no matter how large the batch, calculate their formulas in percentages and use metric weight measurements. That means weighing out each ingredient, even if it is a liquid, and notating the weight in grams.

Since our ingredient quantities are not measured out in grams but instead provided in an approximated liquid equivalent (teaspoons and tablespoons), the yields of our recipes are approximate and you may notice that they vary slightly from the amounts you produce.

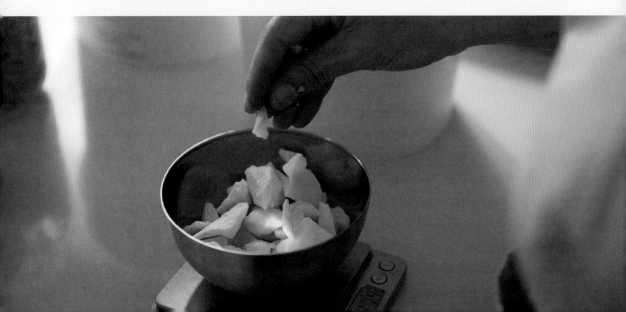

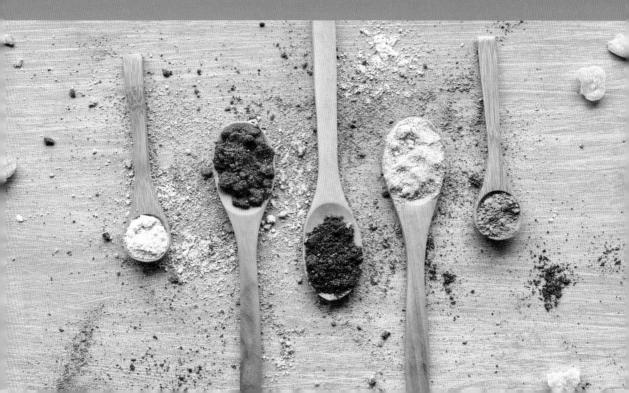

Part 2
BEAUTY RECIPES

FACIAL CARE

Moisturizers

Special Treatments

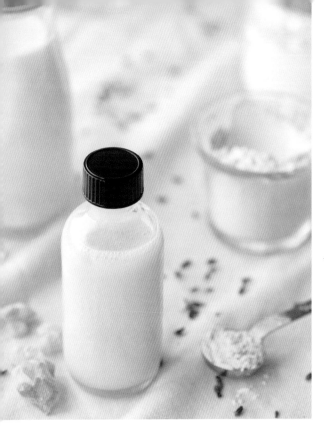

ALMOND MILK FACIAL CLEANSER

- glass measuring pitcher
- small stainless steel whisk
- 1 (1-ounce) amber glass or non-BPA plastic bottle with a flip-top or pump dispenser

---

- **2 teaspoons vegetable glycerin**
- **⅛ teaspoon xanthan gum**
- **1 teaspoon tapioca starch**
- **1 teaspoon castile soap**
- **2 tablespoons almond milk**
- **1 drop vitamin E**
- **10 drops Soothing Mask Essential Oil Synergy (see page 51)**

10 MINUTES

1 FLUID OUNCE

Facial cleansing is an important twice-a-day ritual to rid the skin's surface of impurities and ensure its overall health and balance. After all, our skin is exposed to dirt, pollution, bacteria, and viruses, plus the buildup of dead skin cells, on a daily basis. Cleansing is especially critical at night, when the skin requires oxygen to repair itself. But don't discount a morning cleanse—it works wonders by removing dead skin cells that accumulate overnight as well as allergens (such as dust) that make their way onto your skin through air-conditioning or heating systems.[1] Also, don't forget that cleansing provides a clean slate for applying nourishing moisturizers.[2]

Almond milk is a superfood that is especially useful for aging, dry, and sensitive skin. This under-celebrated topical ingredient contains antioxidants that work to keep skin protected against free radicals and also boasts vitamin B2, which helps preserve healthy tissues, support circulation, and enhance hydration.[3] On top of all that, almond milk contains essential fatty acids, which we all need to maintain moisture and keep our skin balanced.[4]

STEPS

1. Pour the vegetable glycerin into a glass measuring pitcher.

2. Sprinkle in the xanthan gum and begin whisking vigorously. Whisk for 3 minutes nonstop, making sure the xanthan gum dissolves completely into the vegetable glycerin.

3. While continuing to whisk, sprinkle in the tapioca starch and continue to whisk for another minute until fully combined.

4. Slowly drizzle in the castile soap, being mindful not to raise any foam. Keep whisking for another 2 minutes, until the ingredients are well combined.

5. As you continue slowly whisking, drizzle in the almond milk and whisk for another 2 to 3 minutes. You will notice the consistency beginning to slightly thicken.

6. Add the vitamin E and synergy and continue to whisk until all the ingredients are well blended.

7. Pour the product into the bottle and cap tightly. We strongly recommend using this cleanser within 1 week, since the almond milk is perishable. The cleanser should not separate, but if it does, just give it a gentle shake before use. Keep refrigerated to extend the shelf life beyond 1 week.

Beauty Note!

An almond milk cleanser can be blended in about 10 minutes, but if you make almond milk from scratch (highly recommended; see the recipe on page 158), you will need to kick things off 8 to 10 hours in advance, since the almonds need to soak before you can create the milk.

Beauty Note!

Since we are using xanthan gum as one of our ingredients, we need to follow a very precise procedure to blend everything together to ensure the quality of the final product.

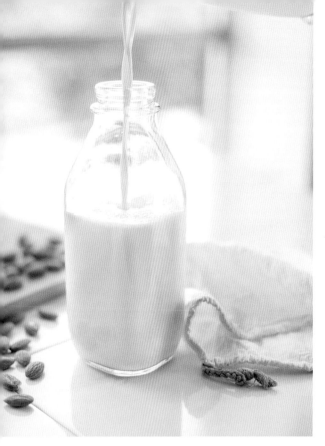

FRESH HOMEMADE ALMOND MILK

- *2 large glass or ceramic bowls*
- *standard (40-ounce) blender*
- *nut milk bag*
- *1 container with a lid*

- *1 cup raw almonds*
- *6 cups spring water, divided*

8 TO 10 HOURS FOR SOAKING THE ALMONDS; 10 MINUTES FOR MAKING THE ALMOND MILK

3 1/2 CUPS

STEPS

1. Place the almonds in a glass or ceramic bowl and add 2½ cups of the spring water. Soak the almonds for 8 to 10 hours.

2. Drain the almonds, discard the soaking water, and transfer the almonds to a blender with the remaining 3½ cups spring water. Blend on high for about 90 seconds.

3. Once the almonds are fully incorporated into the water, place the nut milk bag over another large bowl and carefully pour the entire contents of the blender into the bag, allowing the liquid to make its way completely through the cloth and into the bowl. Lightly squeeze the bag so that all the milk makes its way out of the bag.

4. Pour the strained milk into the container, cap tightly, and store in the refrigerator for up to 4 days.

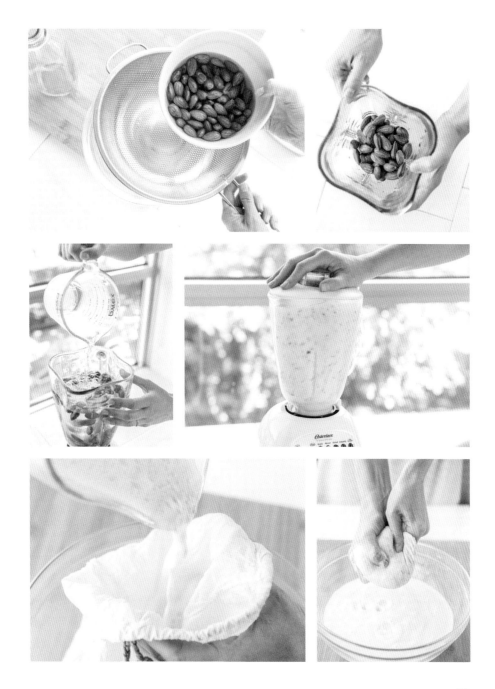

Gums

WHAT THEY ARE

A gum is an ingredient that is used in skin- and body-care formulations to change the viscosity of the product. Simply put, gums are thickeners that help adjust the touch and feel of the recipe. Gums generally are derived from two kinds of sources: (1) natural sources, which include plant-based materials and naturally fermented materials, and (2) synthetic sources, which are laboratory-designed chemicals. Natural gums come from plant resins and secretions, ground seeds and other plant materials, sea plants, or the natural fermentation process of naturally occurring microorganisms. Here are some examples of natural gums:

— xanthan gum

— guar gum

— locust bean gum

— carrageenan gum

— acacia gum

Beauty Tip!

Gums can be finicky to work with, so it is best to follow a specific procedure, like first dissolving them in glycerin or a water like hydrosol. The best results are achieved when gums are used in very small percentages.

HOW THEY ARE USED

Gums are used to make the formula feel a certain way; they add unique textures. You can find them in cleansers, creams, and gels, where they help combine the oil and water components so they don't separate. Gums generally do not have strong therapeutic properties, though they can contribute to soothing and calming the skin.

Preservatives

WHAT THEY ARE

When you are using fresh plant-based botanical ingredients, be mindful that their shelf life is extremely short. Think about preparing our beauty recipes as you would think about cooking a special meal, understanding that the dish is best served immediately and that leftovers lose their potency and flavor and may spoil quickly. And although many of our recipes are intended for immediate use, we feel it is important to bring up the subject of preservatives.

A preservative is either a naturally occurring chemical (like some of the molecules that occur naturally in tea tree essential oil, for example) or a synthetically created chemical that is added to food or body care products to prevent them from decaying, changing chemically over time and becoming contaminated with undesirable microbes that could be harmful to our health.

HOW THEY ARE USED

Preservatives are used to increase the shelf life of a product and prevent contamination. Since our recipes are all intended for immediate use, we do not include any natural preservatives.

We'd like to note that our omission of preservatives in our recipes doesn't mean that we are advocating "preservative-free" products. It's a good practice to be mindful that any plant-based beauty product has the potential to degrade and become contaminated by the growth of yeast, mold, and other possibly harmful microbes. A product that is marketed and sold as "preservative-free" isn't necessarily safer. We see preservatives as playing an important role in keeping natural beauty products safe and stable.

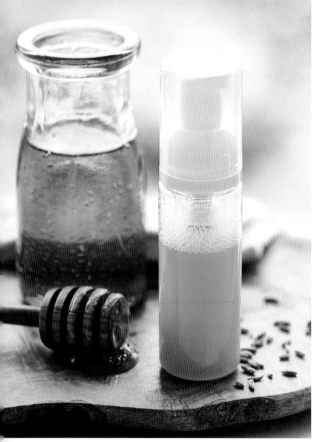

FOAMING HONEY
FACIAL CLEANSER

- *glass bowl or beaker*
- *glass or wooden stirrer*
- *1 (2-ounce) non-BPA plastic bottle with a foaming pump*

- *1 tablespoon honey*
- *1 tablespoon castile soap*
- *1 drop vitamin E*
- *26 drops Foaming Honey Essential Oil Synergy (see page 50)*
- *2 tablespoons distilled water*

10 MINUTES

2 FLUID OUNCES

There is something uniquely luxurious about using a special foaming pump for this cleanser recipe featuring honey. Like a fine dessert, the honey provides a richly nourishing sweetness that soothes both body and soul.

STEPS

1. Pour the honey and castile soap into a glass bowl or beaker and stir until well combined.
2. Continue stirring as you add the vitamin E and synergy.
3. Slowly add the distilled water into the honey and soap mixture and continue stirring until the ingredients are fully incorporated. The color should be a very pale yellow.
4. Transfer the mixture to the bottle and twist the foaming pump into place. The cleanser is ready to use and will stay fresh for about 3 weeks. This recipe is good for all skin types.

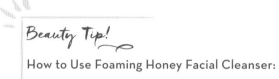

Beauty Tip!

How to Use Foaming Honey Facial Cleanser:

1. *Place one to two full pumps of the cleanser in the palm of your hand.*
2. *Rub your hands together and add water to build up the foam.*
3. *Generously apply the foam to your face, gently making circular motions to cleanse your skin fully.*
4. *After 30 seconds to 1 minute, use warm water to rinse off the cleanser.*
5. *Pat your face dry using a clean cotton towel.*

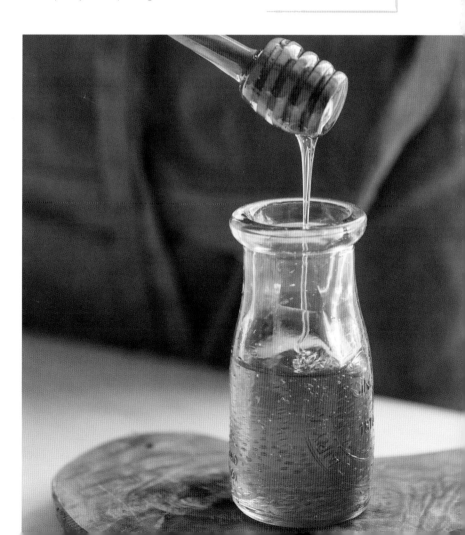

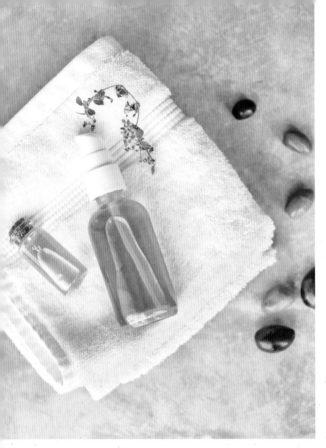

OLIVE OIL FACIAL CLEANSER

- glass or stainless steel bowl or beaker
- glass or wooden stirrer
- 1 (1-ounce) glass bottle or non-BPA plastic bottle with a dropper cap or flip-top

---

- *1 tablespoon plantain-infused olive oil*
- *1 tablespoon sesame oil*
- *1 teaspoon vegetable glycerin*
- *10 drops Olive Oil Cleanser Essential Oil Synergy (see page 50)*

10 MINUTES

1 FLUID OUNCE

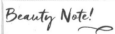

Beauty Note!

Keep in mind that if you are making your own plantain-infused olive oil, you will need to start the process for the infusion 3 months in advance. See page 92 for how to infuse herbal oils.

Oil cleansing is the process of using oil, instead of soap or a cleanser, to dissolve and remove impurities from the skin. It works by massaging extracts from botanicals, vegetables, and fruit into the skin to cleanse pores of dirt and bacteria. These natural ingredients effectively tackle sebum (oil produced by the skin) while nourishing and balancing skin. Olive oil, which plays a starring role in this recipe, is a favorite ingredient due to its antioxidant powers[5] and the presence of vitamin E. We recommend using an extra-virgin olive oil that has been cold-pressed.

STEPS

1. In a glass or stainless steel bowl or beaker, combine the olive oil, sesame oil, and vegetable glycerin, and stir together.
2. Add the synergy and stir gently to combine.

3.   Transfer the mixture to the bottle, fasten the cap, and shake. Store in a cool, dark area. Do not refrigerate. The cleanser should last for 1 year.

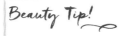

Beauty Tip!

How to Use Olive Oil Facial Cleanser:

You will need two cotton pads and a hydrosol of your choice in a spray bottle.

1. *Lightly dampen the two cotton pads on both sides with the hydrosol.*
2. *Pump two helpings of Olive Oil Facial Cleanser into the center of one side of each dampened pad.*
3. *Using gentle circular motions, start around your nose and cheeks and work your way around your entire face with one of the pads. If you find the pad is quickly absorbing a good deal of dirt and grime, continue with the second fresh pad.*
4. *Once your entire face is cleansed, finish off by rinsing with warm water and patting your face dry with a clean cotton towel.*

HOW TO MAKE POWDERS ⎯⎯⎯⎯⎯

Our mask and scrub recipes include a variety of botanical powders as ingredients. It's easy to purchase already dried and powdered vegetables, fruits, herbs, and grains, and we offer a few reliable sources in our resources section (see page 269) to procure them, but if you are inspired to trace these ingredients back to their sources and create the powders yourself, the process is really quite simple.

What you will need

- dehydrator
- spice grinder or coffee grinder
- silicone brush or small wooden spoon
- glass storage jars with tight-fitting lids
- labels

1. Decide what you want to powder and source the ingredients.

Depending on what therapeutic actions you are looking for, you will reach for different types of plant materials, including fruits, vegetables, herbs, and grains. Once you narrow down what you need, we suggest finding a source for fresh, locally grown vegetables, fruits, and herbs, and collecting at least 8 to 16 ounces.

2. Dehydrate it.

Most home-use dehydrators have recommended instructions for preparing fresh fruits, herbs, and vegetables to be dehydrated. We suggest familiarizing yourself with your particular machine to make sure you understand the most effective ways to use it. Here are a few of our own tips:

— **Berries:** Carefully and thoroughly wash and hand-dry all berries, being careful to remove any damaged berries, stems, leaves, and imperfections. We have had better results when we slice strawberries but leave raspberries and blackberries whole. Raspberries and blackberries should be placed on the dehydrator trays with the hollow side facing down for maximum drying. Blueberries should be quickly blanched to slightly pierce their tough skins, but make sure to dry them well before placing them on the dehydrator trays.

— **Fruits:** Fruits dry best when peeled and thinly sliced. We have found misting the slices with freshly squeezed lemon juice while they are on the trays prevents them from browning.

— **Vegetables:** Carefully wash vegetables and then peel if needed, like for carrots, and chop thinly. Make sure they are thoroughly patted dry of all excess water.

— **Herbs:** For flowers we don't recommend washing, but for leaves like peppermint, basil, tarragon, rosemary, thyme, and so on, we suggest you rinse them gently, pluck them from the stems, remove all imperfections, and pat them dry before placing them on the trays.

Follow the recommended instructions for setting temperature and time. In general, we have found setting the dehydrator between 125 and 135 degrees works best. However, be aware of the climate you are in; a more humid environment will increase drying times, whereas a drier zone may decrease them. We suggest checking in on the progress after 10 to 12 hours to gauge it. To test whether the plant material is sufficiently dried, snap the dried fruit or vegetable and listen for a "crack," indicating it is fully dried with no moisture left.

3. Grind it.

When you are certain the material is dried out, gather it up and start grinding. Using a good-quality electric spice or coffee grinder is key for producing softly textured and beautiful-looking powders. A mortar and pestle also works well, but can be more labor-intensive and may not grind the material uniformly.

4. Jar and label it.

We strongly recommend using only glass to store your powders. Make sure the containers are well cleaned and sterilized. Brush out the powders from the grinder, place in jars, and label with the contents and date. They are now ready for use. We recommend keeping your powders refrigerated so they will stay fresh for a few months.

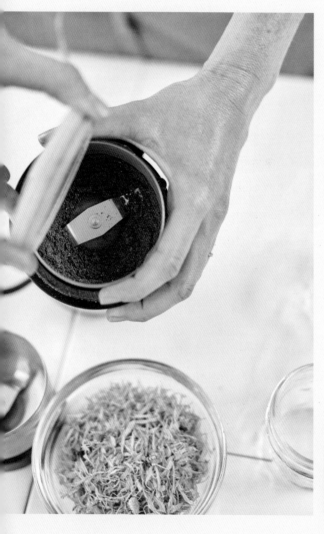

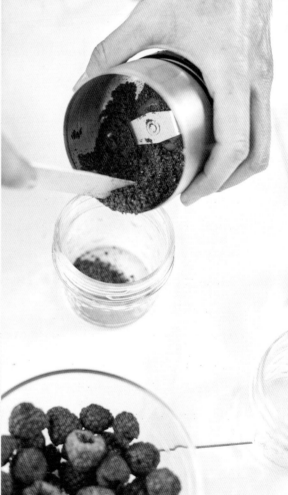

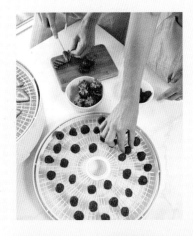
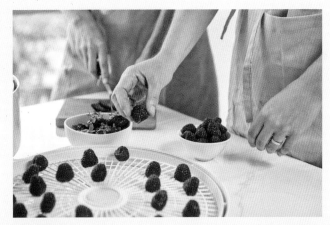
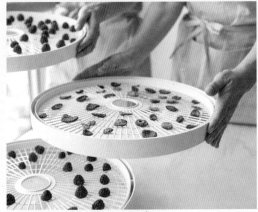
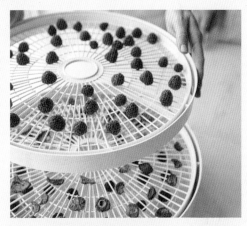
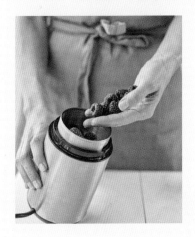
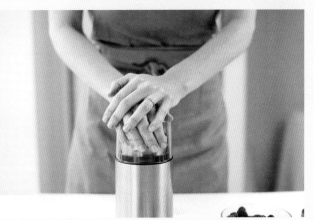

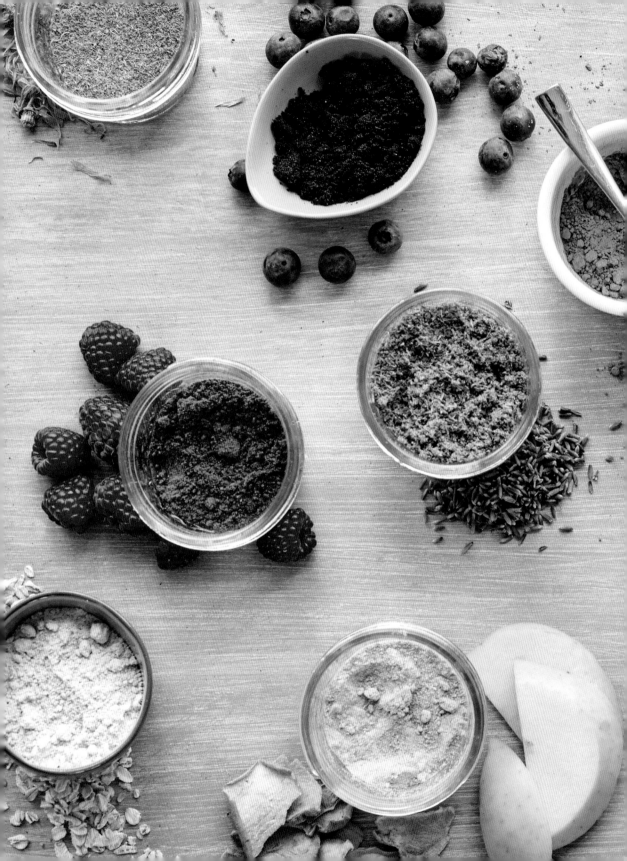

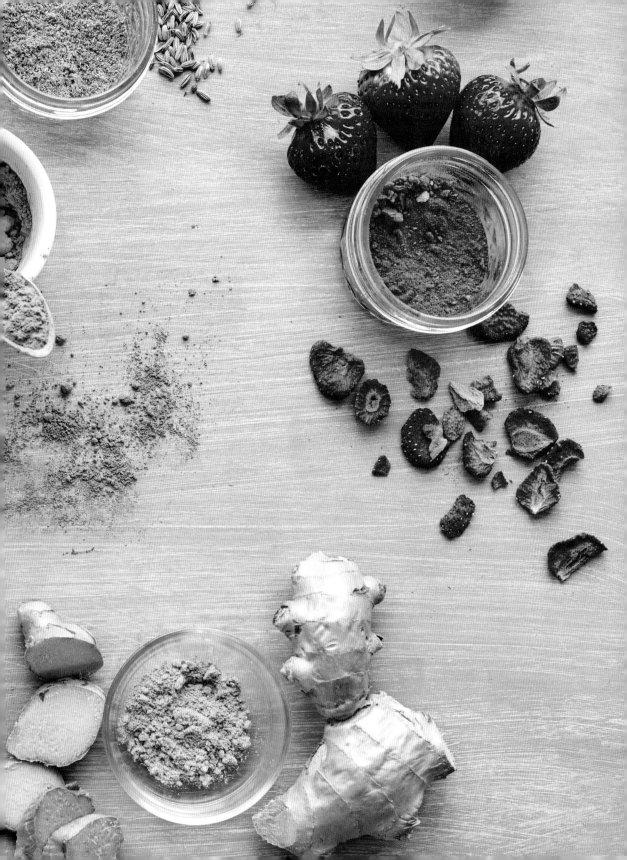

DEEP-CLEANSING FACIAL MASK

- *1 tablespoon bentonite clay powder*
- *1 tablespoon French green clay powder*
- *1/2 teaspoon matcha powder*
- *1/2 teaspoon dried blueberry powder*
- *2 drops Deep-Cleansing Mask Essential Oil Synergy (see page 51)*

Indulging in a facial mask ritual is an excellent way to draw out impurities, improve circulation, and feed your face with needed nutrients. Our Deep-Cleansing Facial Mask is ideal for skin that feels congested, stressed, and dull. We find this formula especially helpful for those who have an oilier complexion or are acne prone.

SOOTHING AND BALANCING FACIAL MASK

- *2 tablespoons rose clay powder*
- *1/2 teaspoon organic apple powder*
- *1/2 teaspoon organic oat flour*
- *2 drops Soothing Mask Essential Oil Synergy (see page 51)*

Our Soothing and Balancing Facial Mask is perfect for skin that is stressed out by seasonal changes, diet shifts, lack of sleep, and hormonal ups and downs.

SENSITIVE FACIAL MASK

- *1 tablespoon plus 1 1/2 teaspoons pink kaolin clay powder*
- *1/2 teaspoon dried calendula flower powder*
- *1/2 teaspoon dried lavender flower powder*
- *1/2 teaspoon organic oat flour*
- *2 drops Sensitive Skin Essential Oil Synergy (see page 51)*

If your skin is especially dry, mature, delicate, and/or generally reactive, this mask made with a plant trio of calendula, lavender, and oats is your new best friend for gently cleansing and drawing out impurities.

- small glass bowl
- glass or wooden stirrer
- 1 (1-ounce) glass jar with a tight-fitting lid

5 MINUTES OR LESS

1 (1-OUNCE) JAR OF DRY POWDERED CLAYS, GOOD FOR 2 USES

STEPS

1. In a small glass bowl, stir together all the dry ingredients until combined, paying close attention to ensure they are fully incorporated.

2. Gently add the synergy. You will notice small liquid droplets forming on the surface of the powders; use a stirrer to break them up and incorporate them into the powdered mixture until they are fully dissipated.

3. Transfer the dry blended ingredients to the glass jar, cap tightly, and give it a gentle shake. The facial mask mixture should stay fresh for 1 month.

Beauty Tip!

How to Use the Facial Mask:

1. Lightly dampen your face with warm water.
2. In a small dish, measure out 1 tablespoon of the facial mask mixture.
3. Add 1 to 1½ teaspoons of warm water or strongly brewed herbal tea, and mix well until the mask forms a loose paste. You may find it necessary to add slightly more water to achieve your desired consistency. Ideally you want to create a mixture with a paste-like consistency that will stay on your face without dripping.
4. Using your fingers, smooth the mask around your chin, cheeks, nose, and forehead, being careful to leave ample space around your eyes, nostrils, and mouth.
5. Sit back and relax. The clays should start to harden in about 5 minutes. Allow yourself 5 to 10 minutes to sit with the mask.
6. Rinse your face with a damp, warm cloth and gently remove the residue until your face is clean.

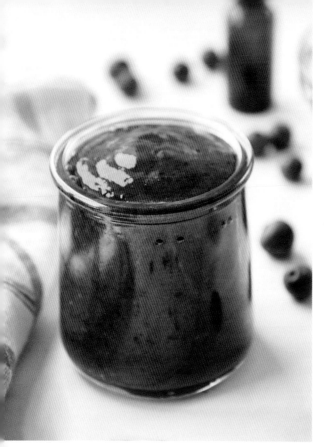

FRESH ENZYME FACIAL MASK

- *standard (40-ounce) blender*
- *small glass or stainless steel bowl*
- *glass or wooden stirrer*

- *1 ounce sugar-free soy yogurt*
- *1 ounce fresh blueberries*
- *1 ounce fresh raspberries*
- *1 drop lavender essential oil*

5 MINUTES OR LESS

1 USE

We paired fresh blueberries and raspberries to double up on the enzyme power in our supercharged healing facial mask that works to repair skin from acne, stress, and exposure to sun and pollution. This super-fresh recipe is for one-time, immediate use.

Beauty Note!

Soy yogurt contains probiotics, which when applied topically can help maintain the balance of your skin's microbiome.

STEPS

1. Place the yogurt, blueberries, and raspberries into a blender, and blend on high for 30 seconds to 1 minute, until the ingredients are partly liquefied.

2. Transfer the mixture to a small glass or stainless steel bowl. Add the lavender essential oil and stir into the mixture.

3. Apply the mask to your face immediately and let it sit for about 10 minutes.

4. Rinse off the mask with warm water and then pat your skin dry with a clean cotton towel.

Beauty Note!

Enzymes are naturally occurring chemicals that living organisms (like plants and animals) produce. They act like catalysts to speed up the rate of other chemical reactions necessary for that organism to survive and can be found in fruits, vegetables, and microorganisms that are used to ferment yogurt, wine, and cheese. Enzymes are incredibly useful in skincare, especially when you are seeking to exfoliate or protect skin from oxidative damage.[6] They can also speed up the process of exfoliation, reduce inflammation, and even out skin tone.

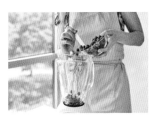
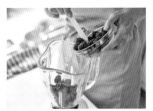
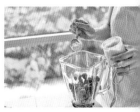

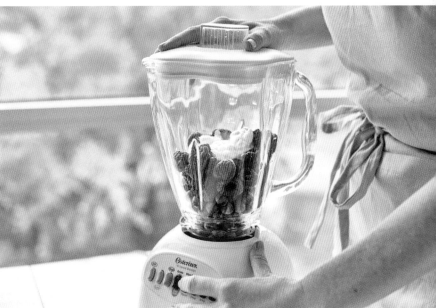

Microbiome

The skin is our largest organ and has several functions that are integral to our overall health. One function is to act as a barrier and to prevent potentially harmful and destructive pathogens from entering our bodies. In order to do this, the skin creates a kind of film that coats the entire surface of the epidermis (the top layer of our skin). This film, also known as the acid mantle, is a complex mixture of our own natural oils (sebum), sweat, and naturally occurring microbes. Recent studies[7] have documented that this unique ecosystem has a profound impact on the health of not only our skin but also our whole body.[8]

Researching and studying the skin's microbiome is becoming a fast-growing field,[9] and new skin and body care products are emerging that address ways to balance and support the millions of bacteria that live on our skin's surface.[10]

That is why we have decided to include yogurt in our Fresh Enzyme Facial Mask (page 174). By reintroducing live cultures and bacteria into our skin's ecosystem, we can help reduce inflammation, boost immunity, and soothe irritation.[11]

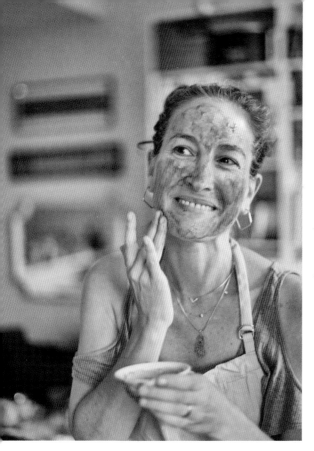

FRESH ANTI-INFLAMMATORY AND BRIGHTENING FACIAL MASK

- standard (40-ounce) blender
- small glass bowl
- glass or wooden stirrer

- 4 ripe strawberries
- 1 tablespoon honey
- 1 drop German (blue) chamomile essential oil

1 USE

5 MINUTES OR LESS

This simple, natural, and *fresh* three-ingredient mask is especially helpful for dull skin needing a life lift or skin prone to acne breakouts. With the healing qualities of honey, the brightening power of strawberries, and the anti-inflammatory benefits of chamomile, you don't have to look past your kitchen cabinet to blend a mask that will leave your skin radiating health and happiness.

Beauty Note!

Did you know using fresh strawberries helps brighten up those pesky dark (age) spots?[12] What a delightful (and affordable) DIY age-delay treatment!

STEPS

1. Place the strawberries and honey into a blender and blend on high for 1 to 2 minutes, until the ingredients are mostly liquefied.

2. Transfer the mixture to a small glass bowl. Add the German chamomile essential oil and stir together until well incorporated.

3.   Apply the mask to your face immediately and let it sit for about 10 minutes.

4.   Rinse off the mask with warm water and pat your skin dry with a clean cotton towel.

Beauty Note!

Not only are strawberries tasty, but they also help cleanse, refresh, and brighten skin, as well as address acne,[13] due to the presence of salicylic acid—an ingredient touted for its ability to unclog pores.[14] Other skin benefits of salicylic acid include removing dead skin cells, reducing puffiness and inflammation, and drawing out toxins. It's also been shown to even out skin tone. All of these are excellent properties when the skin needs a healing boost after an acne breakout.

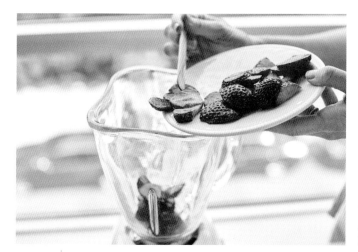
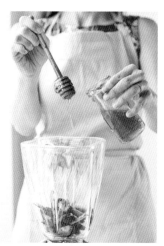
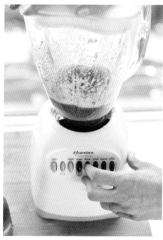
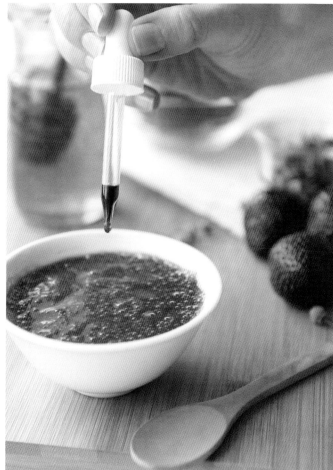
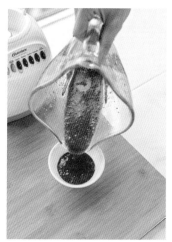

ANTI-AGING FACIAL SCRUB

- *1¹/2 teaspoons organic strawberry powder*
- *1¹/2 teaspoons organic raspberry powder*
- *1¹/2 teaspoons organic apple powder*
- *1¹/2 teaspoons organic oat flour*
- *¹/2 teaspoon matcha powder*
- *8 drops Anti-aging Essential Oil Synergy (see page 51)*

Did you know our skin is designed to naturally exfoliate, meaning once the hardened protein-filled cells of our skin reach the outermost layer, they usually just imperceptibly slough off? This natural process takes about fourteen days when the skin and its complex matrix of oils and fats are working in sync. But often, due to diet, stress, and age, the process can slow down or be thrown off-kilter, making the cells pile up and harden, which is why we may see buildup of dry, flaky facial skin.

To give these cells an extra push, we have designed three plant-based facial scrubs (for varying skin types) that encourage movement and circulation in the lower layers of the epidermis, resulting in rejuvenated, glowing skin.

DETOX FACIAL SCRUB

- *2¹/2 teaspoons chickpea flour*
- *pinch of wheatgrass powder*
- *¹/4 teaspoon turmeric powder*
- *¹/4 teaspoon kale powder*
- *8 drops Detox Essential Oil Synergy (see page 51)*

Our skin, especially our face, is bombarded daily by an assortment of skin and cosmetic products (such as moisturizers, sunscreens, and makeup) and is literally "face first" when navigating all sorts of environmental pathogens. The result? Pores that clog easily, dull skin tone, and discoloration. One of the best ways to encourage the skin to detoxify, increase its vibrancy, and brighten up is to exfoliate using a blend of ingredients that are known to promote circulation and to even skin tone.

BALANCING FACIAL SCRUB

- *1 tablespoon oat flour*
- *1 teaspoon dried calendula flower powder*
- *1 teaspoon dried lavender flower powder*
- *1 teaspoon dried chamomile flower powder*
- *8 drops Balancing Essential Oil Synergy (see page 51)*

We know how challenging it can be to find a facial scrub that won't lead to irritation or reddening. Instead of forgoing exfoliation, which is important for skin regeneration and increased blood flow, for fear of causing a harsh reaction, try this gentle recipe that works wonders and helps skin become less reactive and inflamed.

- small glass bowl
- glass or wooden stirrer
- 1 (1-ounce) glass jar with a tight-fitting lid

5 MINUTES OR LESS

1 (1-OUNCE) JAR OF A DRY POWDERED SCRUB, GOOD FOR ABOUT 3 USES

STEPS

1. In a small glass bowl, combine all the dry ingredients and stir until well incorporated.
2. Gently add the synergy. You will notice small liquid droplets forming on the surface of the dry ingredients; use a stirrer to break them up and incorporate them into the powdered mixture until they are fully dissipated.
3. Transfer the blended ingredients to the glass jar, cap tightly, and give it a gentle shake. It should stay fresh for 1 month.

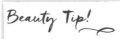

Beauty Tip!

How to Use a Facial Scrub:

1. Dampen your face with warm water.
2. Pour about 2 teaspoons of the dry powdered scrub into the palm of one hand.
3. Add 1 to 1½ teaspoons of warm water and mix well until the scrub forms a loose paste.
4. Apply a fingerful of the wet scrub to your chin, cheeks, and forehead. Rub in a gentle circular motion for 1 to 2 minutes, making sure to cover your entire face but avoiding your eyes, mouth, and nostrils.
5. Rinse your face with warm water and wipe away the remaining residue with a soft wet washcloth until your face is clean.

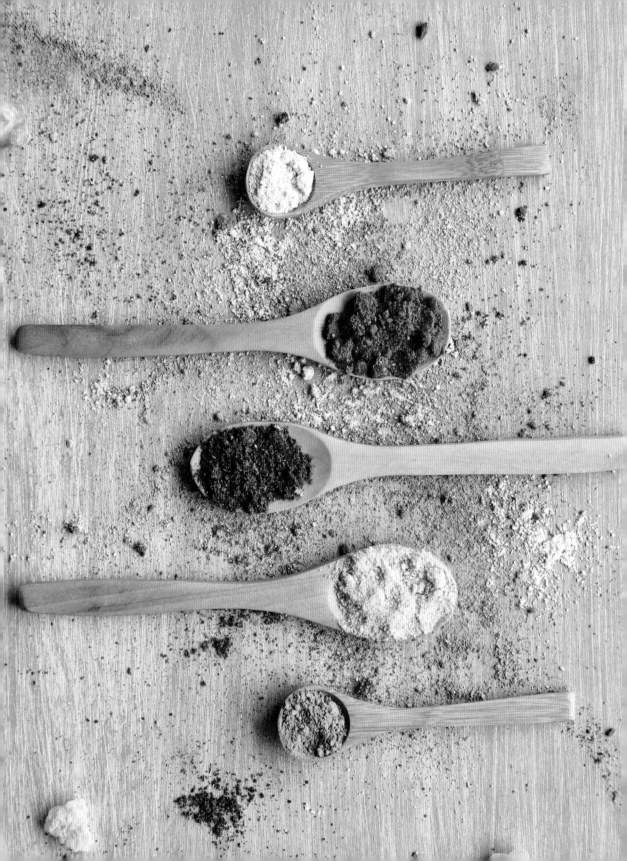

Chlorophyll and Skin Health

Chlorophyll is the green pigment in all green plants that is responsible for helping the plant capture light energy and transform it into chemical energy (photosynthesis). Research has shown that when chlorophyll is applied topically, it can aid in tissue regeneration and healing.[15]

No wonder chlorophyll has become a go-to ingredient for wound healing and anti-aging products. All deep green botanicals, like leafy green vegetables, sea vegetables, and wheatgrass, contain it. We included wheatgrass, matcha, and kale powder in some of our facial scrubs and masks to help deliver these powerful properties directly into our skin. Chlorophyll also has detoxifying and anti-inflammatory effects and is a strong antioxidant.[16]

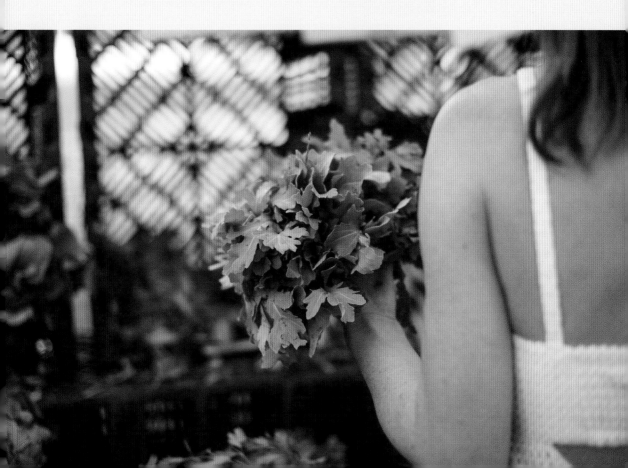

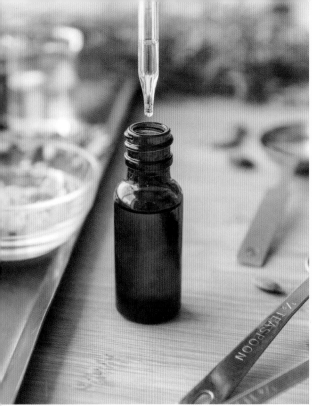

EVENING ANTI-AGING FACIAL SERUM

- small glass beaker
- glass or wooden stirrer
- 1 (1-ounce) amber glass bottle with a dropper cap

- 2 tablespoons apricot kernel oil
- 1½ teaspoons jojoba oil
- 1¼ teaspoons carrot-infused sunflower seed oil (see page 185)
- ½ teaspoon pumpkin seed oil
- ¼ teaspoon sea buckthorn oil
- 10 drops Anti-aging Essential Oil Synergy (see page 52)

10 MINUTES

1 FLUID OUNCE

As we age, the skin's natural production of sebum decreases, which leads to diminished elasticity, dry skin, and the appearance of fine lines. To combat this condition, facial serums offer a natural way to deeply nourish and replenish the skin with essential fatty acids and vitamin-rich reparative oils.

STEPS

1. In a small glass beaker, gently mix all the carrier oils together. The color will be light orange with a hint of light brown; this serum will easily absorb, so don't worry about the color staining your skin.
2. Add the synergy to the carrier oil mixture and continue stirring for about 30 seconds.
3. Once the synergy is nicely incorporated, slowly pour the serum into the glass bottle, fasten the cap, and shake well. Your facial serum is now ready for use and will last for 3 months. Keep in mind that over time the aroma will intensify as the oils blossom into one another.

Beta-carotene, Vitamin A/Retinoids, and Their Effects on Aging

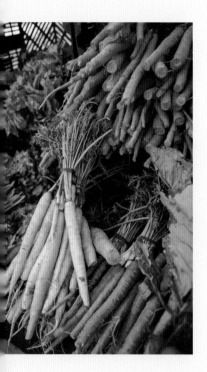

Beta-carotene is the deep orange/red pigment that is found in fresh fruits and vegetables[17] and transforms into vitamin A in our skin and bodies.[18] Vitamin A is required for the proper function of our immune system and our vision; for the growth of our bone tissue; and for the growth, repair, and differentiation of our skin cells.[19] It's also a very strong antioxidant.

Some of the beta-carotene-rich oils we turn to for beauty blending include sea buckthorn oil, tomato seed oil, and carrot-infused sunflower seed oil. The distinctive orange-gold hue of the oil reveals its rich beta-carotene content.[20]

Vitamin A is also known as a class of molecular compounds called retinoids. Chemists have been able to isolate these compounds from naturally occurring sources and infuse them into anti-aging and anti-acne skincare products for their unique ability to support and increase cell regeneration (so you may find retinol listed as an ingredient on its own).

Unfortunately, retinoids, when removed and isolated from plant material and then incorporated on their own as an ingredient in a skincare product, have been shown to make our skin extremely sensitive and vulnerable to environmental damage[21] and potential carcinogens.[22] That's why many clean beauty advocates advise avoiding products that contain them.

What's our take on retinoids? We prefer using whole-plant ingredients that are loaded with naturally occurring beta-carotene instead of incorporating isolated components that have been manipulated in a laboratory. To us, the focus should always be on the whole rather than on an individual molecule or particular chemical component. We feel strongly that the power of beta-carotene to heal wounds and regenerate cells and tissue is remarkable, and whenever possible we will always opt for including the whole, unrefined oils of sea buckthorn, tomato seed, pumpkin seed, and infused carrot root oil into our formulations in order to reap the benefits of retinoids.

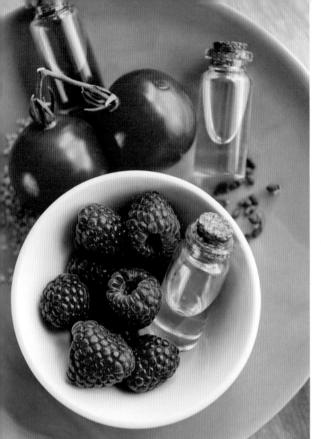

DAY FACIAL OIL FOR BALANCING AND DE-STRESSING SKIN

- *glass measuring pitcher*
- *glass or wooden stirrer*
- *1 (1-ounce) glass or non-BPA plastic bottle with a cap or dropper cap*

- *2½ teaspoons jojoba oil*
- *2½ teaspoons apricot kernel oil*
- *½ teaspoon borage seed oil*
- *½ teaspoon red raspberry seed oil*
- *½ teaspoon tomato seed oil*
- *10 drops Day Facial Oil for Balancing and De-stressing Skin Essential Oil Synergy (see page 52)*

5 MINUTES OR LESS

1 FLUID OUNCE, GOOD FOR ABOUT A DOZEN USES (ONE USE IS ABOUT 1/2 TEASPOON)

Everyday stressors, like seasonal changes, lack of sleep, and pollution, can throw our skin off balance. We can support our skin's natural ability to navigate these obstacles by applying facial oil, which can serve as excellent nourishment and a much-needed layer of protection. It can also help keep our skin even-toned, healthy, and calm.

STEPS

1. In a glass measuring pitcher, combine all the carrier oils together and mix until fully incorporated.
2. Add the synergy and keep mixing.
3. Pour the mixture slowly into the bottle, cap, and shake well. This facial oil will stay fresh for 2 months.

DAY FACIAL OIL FOR BRIGHTENING AND CIRCULATION

- glass measuring pitcher
- glass or wooden stirrer
- 1 (1-ounce) glass or non-BPA plastic bottle with a cap or dropper cap

---

- 2¼ teaspoons jojoba oil
- 2¼ teaspoons apricot kernel oil
- ½ teaspoon yarrow-infused olive oil (see page 92)
- ¾ teaspoon rose hip seed oil
- ¼ teaspoon borage seed oil
- 10 drops Day Facial Oil for Brightening and Circulation Essential Oil Synergy (see page 52)

5 MINUTES OR LESS

1 FLUID OUNCE, GOOD FOR ABOUT A DOZEN USES (ONE USE IS ABOUT 1/2 TEASPOON)

What does it really mean to brighten your skin? We believe it is about encouraging circulation in the tiny capillaries and feeding absorbable nutrients to the delicate layers of our skin. A quick and gentle face massage with our richly nutritive face oil can provide almost immediate results.

We suggest taking a needed time-out with this facial oil to gently massage the face and promote the flow of energy and circulation—you'll see an instant brightening!

STEPS

1. In a glass measuring pitcher, combine all the carrier oils together and mix until fully incorporated.
2. Add the synergy and keep mixing.
3. Pour the mixture slowly into the bottle, cap, and shake well. This face oil will stay fresh for 2 months.

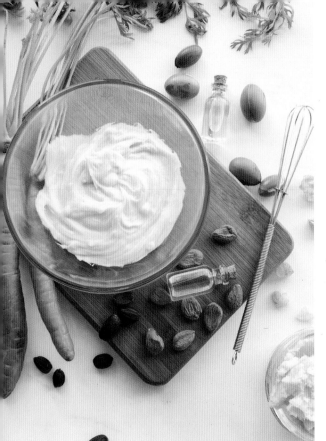

SHEA BUTTER FACE CREAM

- *glass or stainless steel bowl*
- *wooden stick or metal spoon*
- *small stainless steel whisk*
- *1 (2-ounce) glass jar with a tight-fitting lid*

- *2 heaping tablespoons shea butter*
- *1 teaspoon apricot kernel oil*
- *1 teaspoon jojoba oil*
- *1 teaspoon argan oil*
- *6 drops Anti-aging Essential Oil Synergy (see page 52)*

15 MINUTES

2 FLUID OUNCES

We love this face cream year-round but find it especially helpful during the cold, dry months, when our skin becomes parched and cries out for a deeply hydrating and reparative moisturizer. With its soothing and anti-inflammatory properties, it is also a lifesaver after extended exposure to the sun.

STEPS

1. In a glass or stainless steel bowl, mash the shea butter using the back of a spoon or a wooden stick until there are no lumps visible and it is entirely smoothed out.

2. Begin whisking the shea butter until it starts getting creamier.

3. Slowly drizzle in the carrier oils as you continue to whisk the creamed shea butter, until a silky, smooth consistency emerges.

4.   Add the synergy right into the cream and stir together.

5.   Transfer the mixture to the glass jar, cap, and store away from heat. You can use the face cream for 1 month.

Beauty Note!

Shea butter, the starring ingredient in this recipe, offers a beneficial lineup of vitamins A, D, and E, along with fatty acids, making it perfect for facial skin needing some TLC. It is also a celebrated anti-aging ingredient due to its ability to help spur the production of collagen (which helps prevent premature wrinkles and facial lines).[23] Finally, one of our favorite aspects of this beauty ingredient is the presence of cinnamic acid esters, which help protect skin from developing skin tumors potentially caused by UV radiation.[24]

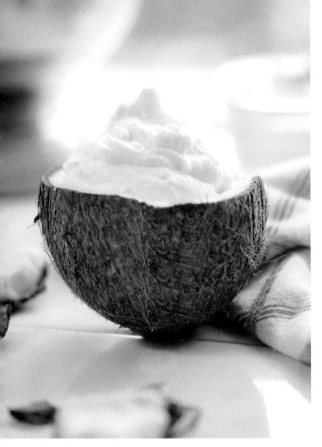

COCONUT WHIP
MAKEUP REMOVER

- food scale
- stand mixer with whip attachment
- spatula
- 1 (2-ounce) glass jar with a tight-fitting lid

- 2 ounces cold, solid organic coconut oil (either raw or naturally deodorized), weighed on a food scale

15 MINUTES

2 OUNCES

This one-ingredient recipe made with coconut oil is a surprisingly simple and healthy alternative to chemical-laden makeup removers. We love the texture, quick-dissolving makeup action, and delicious aroma.

Beauty Note!

Coconut oil solubilizes water-resistant substances (found in many eye shadow and mascara products) and, instead of drying your skin out like many other makeup removers, actually softens your skin.[25]

STEPS

1. Immediately place the cold, solid coconut oil in the bowl of a stand mixer. (It is very important that the coconut oil has not melted down; in order for it to properly fluff up, it must be solid). Whip on high for about 3 minutes.

2. From time to time, stop the mixer to gently scrape the whipped coconut oil down from the sides of the bowl with a spatula and reincorporate it into the center of the mixture.

3. After several minutes, when the coconut oil takes on a fluffy consistency, you will know the process is complete.

4. Transfer the coconut whip with the spatula to the glass jar and cap tightly. Store in a cool place to prevent melting. The makeup remover will last 3 months, if kept out of direct heat.

Beauty Tip!

How to Use Coconut Whip Makeup Remover:

1. *Take a dollop of the coconut whip on your fingertips.*
2. *Apply to your face by softly massaging into all areas where you desire to remove makeup.*
3. *Remove the coconut whip gently with a clean cloth or cotton sheet.*
4. *Follow the makeup removal with a full facial-cleansing routine to avoid clogging pores.*

Beauty Tip!

If the Coconut Whip Makeup Remover hardens over time, don't despair. You can easily warm it up with your hands to soften it before application.

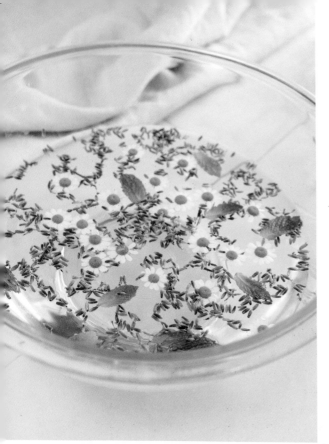

FRESH HERB AND FLOWER FACIAL STEAM

- 1 (1-quart) pot with a lid
- glass or wooden stirrer

- 1 tablespoon fresh or dried lavender flowers
- 1 tablespoon fresh or dried chamomile flowers
- 3 sprigs fresh mint

10 MINUTES

1 USE

Introducing steam (safely) to the skin is an incredibly effective and gentle way to coax out impurities. In this facial steam, we source in-season flowers and herbs bursting with medicinal qualities to enhance the skin-purifying effects of one of our favorite beauty traditions.

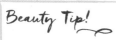

Beauty Tip!

We suggest preparing a gentle facial steam once or twice a week to keep the skin clear and vitalized.

STEPS

1. Fill a pot with 3 to 4 cups of water and bring to a boil.
2. Mix in the flowers and herbs and cover with a lid. Remove from heat.
3. Let the mixture steep for 5 minutes. After your facial steam, discard the water, herbs, and flowers.

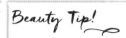

Beauty Tip!

How to Use the Facial Steam:

1. *After your flowers and herbs have steeped for 5 minutes, remove the pot from the stove and set it on a trivet on a tabletop.*
2. *Sit down with the pot in front of you and cover your head with a large towel, creating a kind of tent above the pot.*
3. *Remove the lid and check to see that the steam is not too hot. If it is, wait another 5 minutes.*
4. *Once the temperature feels comfortable, let the scented vapors make their way to your face, being careful not to let the steam get too hot against your skin. Close your eyes and relax, steaming for 5 to 10 minutes.*
5. *When you are finished, splash cool water on your face and gently pat it dry with a clean cotton towel.*

Beauty Note!

The benefits of using steam to promote healthy skin and general well-being are well documented across cultures and throughout the centuries.[26] The gentle warmth and humidity dilate blood vessels to increase the flow of oxygen in the body, which improves circulation and revitalizes cellular health. Steaming also promotes the release of toxins held in the skin and helps the pores open and breathe, encouraging cell regeneration and immunity.

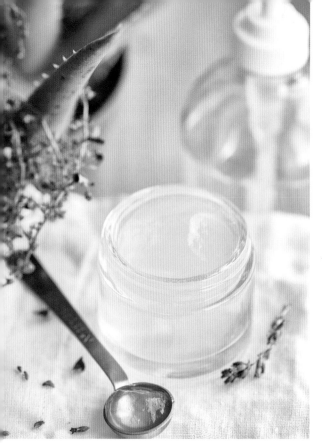

BLEMISH GEL

- small glass or stainless steel bowl or glass beaker
- glass or wooden stirrer
- 1 (1-ounce) glass jar with a tight-fitting lid

- 1 tablespoon plus 2 teaspoons aloe vera gel
- 1 teaspoon witch hazel
- 25 drops Blemish Gel Essential Oil Synergy (see page 53)

5 MINUTES

1 FLUID OUNCE

When unsightly acne appears, we recommend treating it naturally with ingredients that offer antimicrobial, antifungal, and antiseptic properties, along with soothing agents to ensure the inflamed skin does not dry out and become unbalanced. Our blemish gel is packed with healing plant-based essential oils that go right to work on your problem area, while benefiting from a moisturizing and anti-inflammatory base of aloe vera and a cleansing boost of witch hazel.

STEPS

1. In a bowl or beaker, combine the aloe vera and witch hazel.
2. Add the synergy and gently stir together for about 30 seconds, ensuring all the ingredients are fully incorporated.

3. Transfer the blended product to the glass jar and cap tightly. Store in the refrigerator. The blemish gel will stay fresh for 1 month.

Beauty Tips!

How to Use Blemish Gel:

1. Cleanse and tone your skin to create a clean surface.
2. Apply a small drop of the blemish gel directly onto the affected area with your clean fingertip.
3. Leave the gel on and let it fully absorb into your skin.
4. Repeat twice daily or as needed.

Beauty Note!

Aloe has been used for over two thousand years[27] and is often called the "miracle plant" due to its skin-healing powers. It contains a compound called saponin that boasts anti-inflammatory and antibacterial properties,[28] and is prized for its antiseptic powers, moisturizing abilities, and skin-soothing properties.[29]

Recent studies have recognized that aloe also works to improve collagen formation during wound healing,[30] thereby making it a favored acne treatment ingredient.

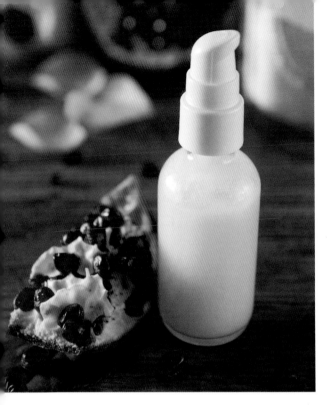

EYE GEL

- 1 (1-cup) glass measuring pitcher
- stainless steel mini whisk
- 1 (1-ounce) glass bottle with a pump dispenser or dropper cap

---

- 1 teaspoon vegetable glycerin
- ⅛ teaspoon xanthan gum
- 1 teaspoon pomegranate seed oil
- 2 tablespoons rose hydrosol

10 MINUTES

1 FLUID OUNCE

Eye gel helps soothe puffy and irritated skin around the eyes and works best when applied right after cleansing in the morning, before moisturizing. We find that it is also helpful when the eye area is feeling itchy and swollen, from allergies or long hours staring at a screen.

STEPS

1. Pour the vegetable glycerin into a glass measuring pitcher, slowly sprinkle in the xanthan gum, and begin whisking together. Whisk vigorously, making sure the xanthan gum dissolves entirely, for about 3 minutes.

2. Slowly add the pomegranate seed oil and continue whisking vigorously until the mixture begins to thicken slightly and the oil is thoroughly incorporated. This could take another 3 minutes of vigorous whisking action.

3. Very slowly drizzle in the rose hydrosol, continuing to whisk until all the hydrosol has been added, about

4 minutes. The gel should begin to look whitish, thicken slightly (developing the consistency of a very thin yogurt), and feel slightly tacky.

4.   Pour the gel into the glass bottle and cap. The eye gel will only last a couple of days. Make sure to keep it refrigerated.

Beauty Tips!

We don't advise incorporating essential oils into your eye gels, since they can be too strong for use on the delicate skin under the eyes. Instead, we like using hydrosols for their cooling and soothing properties and light scents. Try to experiment with different soothing hydrosols and fixed oils.

Beauty Tips!

How to Use Eye Gel:

1. *Pump or drop out an amount of gel about half the size of a dime.*
2. *Gently dab the gel under one of your eyes, being careful not to get it too close to your eye. Repeat for your other eye. Pat gently under your eyes and let the gel dry before moisturizing or adding makeup.*

Beauty Note!

Be sure to refrigerate the eye gel and keep the pump tightly in place. But please be mindful that since we have not added a preservative to this recipe, it will only stay microbe-free for a couple of days. If small dark spots develop on the gel surface, you should discard the gel immediately.

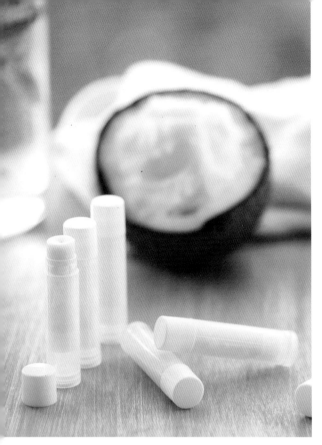

CHOC-O-MINT LIP BALM

- ° *double boiler*
- ° *glass measuring pitcher*
- ° *glass or wooden stirrer*
- ° *18 (0.15-ounce) lip balm tubes*
- ° *parchment paper*

- ° *¼ cup cocoa butter*
- ° *¼ cup beeswax*
- ° *¼ cup coconut oil*
- ° *20 drops peppermint essential oil*

20 MINUTES

18 (0.15-OUNCE) TUBES OF LIP BALM

Unlike the rest of your face, the skin on your lips is extra thin and is devoid of oil glands. As a result, lips can become dehydrated very easily.[31] Therefore, regular moisturizing (with natural balm) is a great way to keep your lips healthy and hydrated. We developed a delicious lip balm recipe with four simple ingredients and a chocolate-mint aroma.

STEPS

1. To set up the double boiler, pour 2 to 3 inches of water into the bottom pot and about 1 inch of water into the upper pot. Heat until the water in the top pot is steaming.

2. Add the cocoa butter, beeswax, and coconut oil to a glass measuring pitcher, and gently place the pitcher into the steaming water of the upper pot. Stir the ingredients continually until they are fully melted.

3. Once the contents of the measuring pitcher are melted and combined, remove the pitcher from the warm water and carefully dry the outside of the pitcher with a paper towel.

4. Add the peppermint essential oil to the mixture and stir.

5. Line up the lip balm tubes on a sheet of parchment paper. With a steady hand, carefully pour the mixture directly from the measuring pitcher into each tube, filling it all the way to the rim. Be sure to do this step right away, while the mixture is hot and fully melted. If the mixture starts to cool (you will know because it will begin setting and will be difficult to work with), simply place the measuring pitcher back into the hot water in the upper pot to remelt the gel. The lip balm will stay fresh for 3 months.

Beauty Note!

Cocoa butter is the main ingredient in chocolate, but did you know it is also a dream for your skin? Cocoa butter is a natural fat extracted from the cacao bean that contains a high concentration of fatty acids, offering lasting hydration and protection from free radicals.[32]

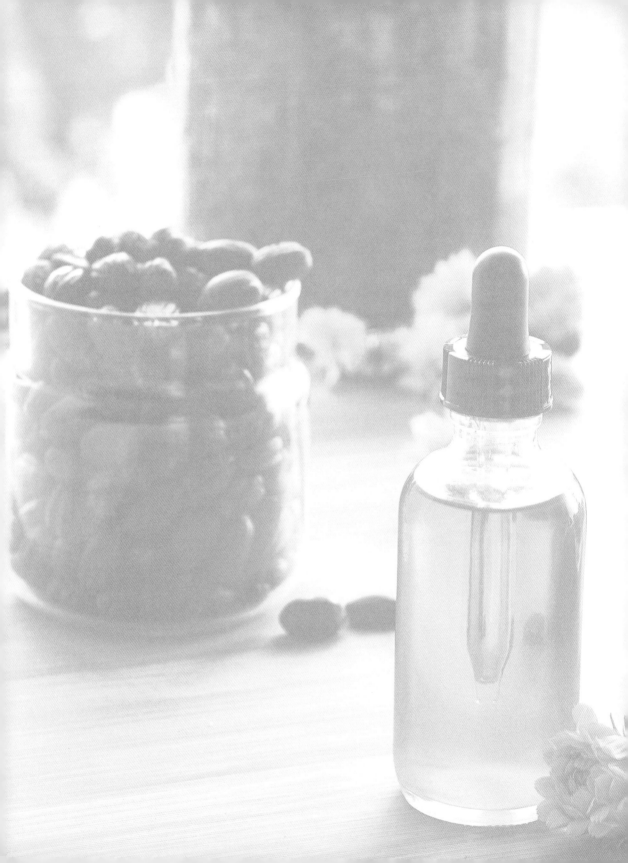

HAIR CARE

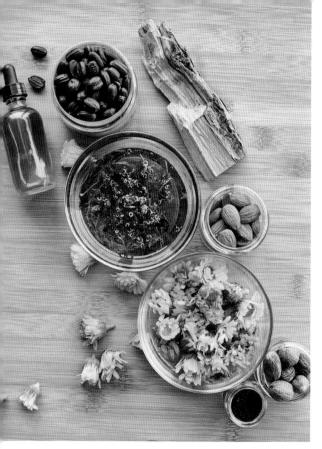

HEALING SCALP SERUM

- glass bowl or beaker
- glass or wooden stirrer
- 1 (2-ounce) amber glass bottle with a dropper cap

- 1 tablespoon jojoba oil
- 1 teaspoon calendula-infused olive oil (see page 92)
- 1 teaspoon almond oil
- 1 teaspoon black cumin seed oil
- 8 drops Healing Scalp Serum Essential Oil Synergy (see page 52)

5 TO 10 MINUTES

2 FLUID OUNCES,

GOOD FOR 1 TO 2

USES

When your scalp feels irritated, dry, or just in need of some TLC, scalp serum made with healing nut, seed, and essential oils is the perfect remedy. Our recipe includes calendula-infused olive oil—a deeply hydrating flower infusion famous for its ability to soothe and heal skin, including dry skin and flaky skin found on the scalp. Also playing a starring role in the blend is black cumin seed oil, which is known for reducing inflammation and improving the speed of healing.[1]

STEPS

1. Combine all the carrier oils in a glass bowl or beaker and stir until fully incorporated. The oil should be a light golden color.

2. Add the synergy and continue to stir until fully incorporated, about 20 seconds.

3.   Transfer the mixture to the glass bottle and shake. The serum is now ready for use and will last for 2 months.

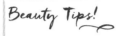

How to Use Scalp Serum:

1. *Start out by applying a generous helping (about 2 tablespoons) onto the palm of your hand and massage onto your dry scalp for about 5 minutes.*
2. *Cover your head—you can either wrap your hair in a dry, heated towel or cover your hair and head with a shower or wool cap.*
3. *Let the serum sit for about 15 minutes to allow the oils to penetrate.*
4. *Take a hot shower and rinse and shampoo your hair. Try to use a gentle shampoo that won't irritate your scalp; we suggest looking for one that doesn't include sulfates (sodium lauryl sulfate or sodium laureth sulfate).*

VITAMIN-RICH HAIR HEALTH SERUM

- glass bowl or beaker
- glass or wooden stirrer
- 1 (1-ounce) amber glass bottle with a dropper cap

- 1 tablespoon jojoba oil
- 1 teaspoon calendula-infused olive oil (see page 92)
- 1 teaspoon almond oil
- 1 teaspoon broccoli seed oil
- 8 drops Healthy Scalp Serum Essential Oil Synergy (see page 52)

5 TO 10 MINUTES

2 FLUID OUNCES,

GOOD FOR 1 TO 2

USES

We all know that broccoli is "good for us," but did you know that this green vegetable also produces specialty seed oil that is rich in vitamins A, C, and K2[2] and ideal for maintaining scalp health? And as far as your hair is concerned, broccoli seed oil also contains calcium, which helps strengthen hair follicles and promote hair growth.[3]

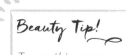

Beauty Tip!

To use this serum, follow the instructions on page 203.

STEPS

1. Combine all the carrier oils in a glass bowl or beaker and stir until fully incorporated. The oil should have a very pale green hue.

2. Add the synergy and continue to stir until fully incorporated, about 20 seconds.

3. Transfer the mixture to the glass bottle and shake. The serum is now ready for use and will last 2 months.

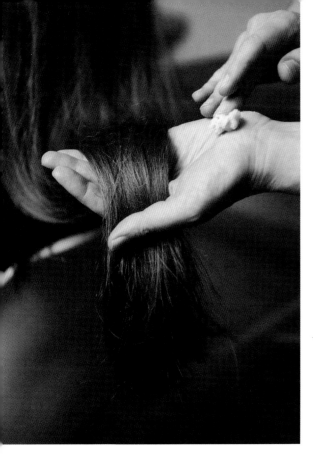

HAIR POMADE

- *double boiler*
- *2 glass measuring pitchers*
- *small stainless steel whisk*
- *stand mixer or handheld mixer, with a whisk attachment*
- *silicone spatula*
- *glass or wooden stirrer*
- *2 or 3 (2-ounce) glass jars with tight-fitting lids*

- *2 tablespoons beeswax pastilles*
- *3 tablespoons shea butter*
- *2 tablespoons jojoba oil*
- *1 tablespoon tapioca starch*
- *20 drops Seductive Massage Essential Oil Synergy (see page 52)*

20 MINUTES

2 OR

3 (2-OUNCE)

JARS

Need to smooth out some flyaway frizz? Or to condition over-processed hair? Feed your locks nutrient-rich, plant-based ingredients with deeply hydrating and reparative hair pomade. Pomade is similar to hair gel or conditioner. It helps style, smooth, and add shine to tired, dull locks.

STEPS

1. To set up the double boiler, pour about 1 inch of water into the bottom pot and about 1 inch of water into the upper pot. Turn the heat on medium to begin warming up the water in both the lower and upper pots.

2. Once the water begins to steam a bit, add the beeswax pastilles and shea butter to the first glass measuring pitcher and place it gently into the upper pot. Keep watch as the ingredients begin to melt. Stir occasionally.

3. Add the jojoba oil to the second glass measuring pitcher and slowly sprinkle in the tapioca starch. Whisk together slowly, making sure the tapioca starch fully dissolves.

4. Once the jojoba and tapioca mixture is fully blended, carefully pour it into the melted beeswax and shea butter, and mix well.

5. Gently lift the warm measuring pitcher out of the top pot of the double boiler, and carefully dry the outside of the pitcher with a paper towel.

6. Pour the melted mixture into the glass or metal bowl you use with your stand or handheld mixer, and let the bowl cool for about 10 minutes.

7. Touch the side of the bowl to test the temperature. When it is no longer too hot to touch but still feels comfortably warm, whip the mixture on high for 3 minutes using the mixer's whisk attachment.

8. Pause the mixer and use a silicone spatula to scrape the mixture down from the sides of the bowl. Whip for another 1 to 2 minutes, until the butter starts to look very thick and creamy.

9. Scrape off as much pomade as possible from the whisk attachment. If you are using a stand mixer, remove the bowl from the mixer.

10. Add the synergy and combine well using the spatula.

11. Portion the pomade into the glass jars and cap tightly. The pomade will last for 3 months.

Beauty Note!

Nourishing hair-styling products are often challenging to find because many are loaded with plasticizers and other petroleum derivatives that, while contributing to shine and hold, expose us to potentially harmful compounds. Our hair conveys a great deal about our health, so when we can feed it whole-plant components, it grows and strengthens.

Beauty Tips!

How to Use Hair Pomade:

1. *Scoop out about 1 teaspoon of the pomade and rub lightly between your hands.*
2. *Gently glide your hands over your hair, paying extra attention to the ends. At this point you can sculpt some waves, smooth out frizzies, and add shine. The pomade can stay in all day and can easily be washed out in your next shampoo.*

Beauty Note!

For gentlemen: *This pomade also works very well for beards and mustaches. Simply rub a small amount of pomade between your hands and glide your hands over your facial hair to smooth and add shape and shine. And if you wish to try your hand at customization, try adjusting the synergy to create an especially pleasing aroma.*

BODY CARE

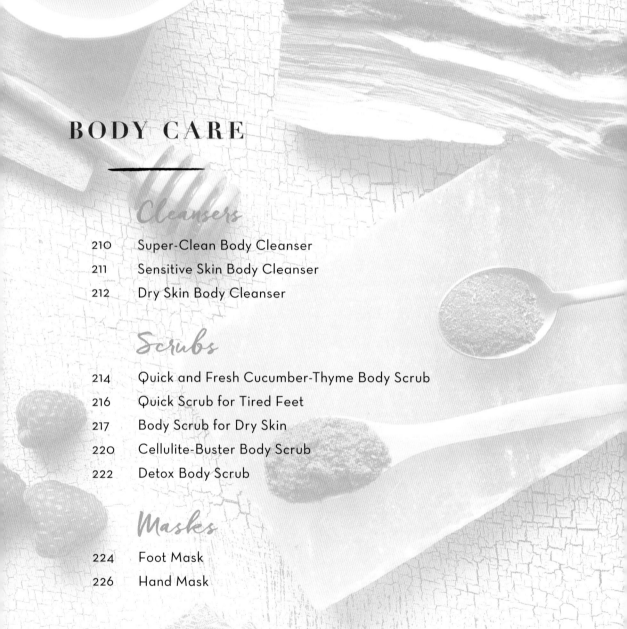

Moisturizers

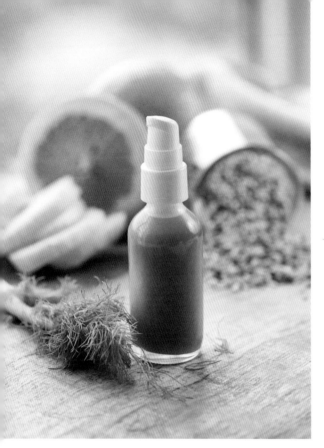

SUPER-CLEAN BODY CLEANSER

- glass measuring pitcher
- glass or wooden stirrer
- 1 (2-ounce) glass or non-BPA plastic bottle with a cap

- 2 tablespoons unscented castile soap
- 2 teaspoons vegetable glycerin
- 2 teaspoons distilled water
- 2 teaspoons organic rice bran powder
- 40 drops Cellulite-Buster Essential Oil Synergy (see page 51)

5 MINUTES OR LESS

2 FLUID OUNCES

What's unique about this particular cleanser? It includes rice bran. Rice bran's gently scrubby texture and rich natural constituents support our skin's own healthy cycle of regeneration.

STEPS

1. In a glass measuring pitcher, combine the castile soap and vegetable glycerin and mix together until fully incorporated.
2. Slowly drizzle in the distilled water and mix well until fully incorporated.
3. Add the rice bran powder and continue stirring.
4. Add the synergy and mix for a couple of seconds.
5. Slowly transfer the mixture to the bottle, cap, and shake well. The cleanser should last for 1 month.

SENSITIVE SKIN BODY CLEANSER

- glass measuring pitcher
- glass or wooden stirrer
- small stainless steel whisk
- 1 (2-ounce) glass or non-BPA bottle with a cap

- 1½ teaspoons vegetable glycerin
- 1½ teaspoons honey
- 1½ teaspoons unscented castile soap
- 1½ teaspoons almond milk
- 30 drops Sensitive Skin Essential Oil Synergy (see page 51)

5 MINUTES OR

LESS

2 FLUID OUNCES,

GOOD FOR

ABOUT 2 USES

If you have sensitive skin, cleansing can be made simple if you start with castile soap and layer your recipe with vegetable oils loaded with essential fatty acids and nutrients. Although castile soap can be drying, its unique chemistry allows it to combine easily with nut and seed oils; the resulting blend offers not only a lovely smooth and silky texture but also a soothing softness to support reactive skin.

STEPS

1. In a glass measuring pitcher, whisk the vegetable glycerin and honey together for about 1 minute.
2. Slowly drizzle in the castile soap, combining it into the mixture with a stirrer.
3. Slowly drizzle in the almond milk, continuing to whisk gently the entire time.
4. Once the mixture looks fully blended, add the synergy and keep stirring.
5. Slowly transfer the mixture to the bottle, cap, and shake well. The cleanser should last for 4 days.

DRY SKIN BODY CLEANSER

- *glass measuring pitcher*
- *glass or wooden stirrer*
- *1 (2-ounce) glass or non-BPA plastic bottle with a cap*

- *1 tablespoon calendula-infused olive oil (see page 92)*
- *3/4 teaspoon honey*
- *2 tablespoons castile soap*
- *2 1/4 teaspoons distilled water*
- *40 drops Dry Skin Essential Oil Synergy (see page 51)*

5 MINUTES OR LESS

2 FLUID OUNCES, GOOD FOR ABOUT 2 USES

If you suffer from dry skin, finding a body cleanser that doesn't further dry and irritate your skin can be a big challenge. Most body washes contain foaming agents that are known to disrupt our skin's pH balance and make us more susceptible to irritation and dryness. A sure way to avoid this is to reach for a cleanser that incorporates ingredients that not only help lift and wash dirt and bacteria away but also support and rebalance our skin's naturally occurring oils.

STEPS

1. In a glass measuring pitcher, combine the calendula-infused olive oil and honey until fully incorporated.
2. Add the castile soap, stirring slowly to avoid foaming.
3. Add the distilled water and continue stirring.
4. Once the mixture looks fully blended, add the synergy and stir to combine.
5. Transfer the mixture to the bottle, cap, and shake well. The cleanser should last for 2 months.

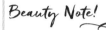

Beauty Note!

Did you know that authentic castile soap is made up of only 100 percent extra-virgin olive oil? It possesses a high percentage of essential fatty acids, specifically oleic acid, and other components that mimic the skin's own chemistry.

The origins of castile soap harken back to the Middle Ages in the Castile area of Spain, where the practice of making soap without the use of tallow (animal fat) began. Castile was known for its abundance of olive oil during this period, and local soap makers used olive oil instead of animal fats and quickly became recognized as producers of high-quality soap. Today, castile soap has come to mean liquid soap made from olive oil and other vegetable fats like coconut oil.

QUICK AND FRESH CUCUMBER-THYME BODY SCRUB

- *standard (40-ounce) blender*
- *glass or stainless steel bowl*
- *glass or wooden stirrer*

- *1 seedless cucumber (we love the Persian variety, but any seedless fresh cucumber will do), peeled and coarsely chopped*
- *1 small bunch fresh tarragon, stems and tiny branches removed*
- *1 small bunch fresh thyme, stems and tiny branches removed*
- *4 tablespoons Dead Sea salt*
- *2 drops rosemary or peppermint essential oil*

5 TO 10 MINUTES

1 USE

Exfoliating your skin is more important than you may think. As you age, cell regeneration (shedding of old skin so new skin can emerge) slows down, and as old skin piles up, your skin starts to appear dry and dull. To avoid this predicament and to help radiant skin emerge, it is essential to exfoliate.

STEPS

1. Place the cucumber, tarragon, and thyme into a blender. Pulsate for 1 to 2 minutes, until the ingredients form a liquid, frothy texture.
2. Transfer the mixture to a glass or stainless steel bowl.
3. Add the Dead Sea salt and stir until fully incorporated.
4. Add the rosemary or peppermint essential oil and mix. Use the scrub immediately.

Beauty Note!

Dead Sea salt contains a plethora of minerals, including magnesium, potassium, and calcium, known to stimulate blood circulation[1] and aid in the process of detoxification.[2]

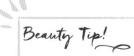

Beauty Tip!

How to Use the Body Scrub:

1. *Take 1 heaping tablespoon of the scrub and apply with your hands or a washcloth to the desired area.*

2. *Use a gentle circular motion for about 1 minute. A light touch is all you will need to effectively cleanse and scrub away dead cells. We recommend exfoliating about once a week.*

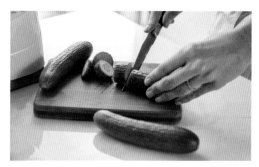
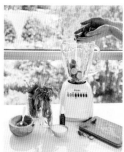
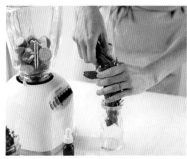
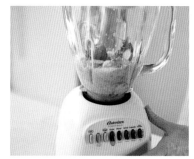
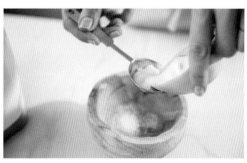
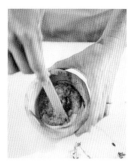

QUICK SCRUB FOR TIRED FEET

- *small glass bowl or beaker*
- *glass or wooden stirrer*
- *1 (2-ounce) glass jar with a tight-fitting lid*

- *2 tablespoons organic sugar*
- *2 teaspoons mustard seed powder*
- *3 teaspoons unscented castile soap*
- *10 drops Tired Feet Essential Oil Synergy (see page 51)*

5 MINUTES OR LESS

2 FLUID OUNCES

Do you neglect your feet? It's easy to forget how important they are to our overall health and well-being. With this in mind, we created an invigorating sugar scrub to scour away stress along with the excess dry skin that can build up over time. The simple act of rubbing our feet can increase blood flow, release muscle tension, and improve our overall health.

STEPS

1. In a small glass bowl or beaker, mix the sugar and mustard seed powder together until well combined.
2. Mix while slowly drizzling in the castile soap until the mixture becomes doughy and creamy looking.
3. Add the synergy and stir well.
4. Transfer the mixture to the glass jar and tightly cap. The scrub will last for 1 month.

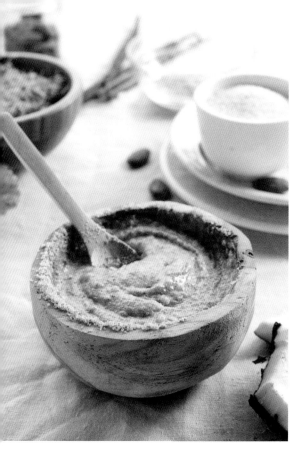

BODY SCRUB FOR DRY SKIN

- *2 small glass bowls*
- *glass or wooden stirrer*
- *stainless steel spoon*
- *small stainless steel whisk*
- *1 (1-ounce) glass jar with a tight-fitting lid*

- *1 tablespoon organic sugar*
- *2 teaspoons finely ground almond meal or almond flour*
- *1 teaspoon dried calendula flower powder*
- *2 teaspoons shea butter (either unrefined or naturally deodorized)*
- *2 teaspoons coconut oil, naturally deodorized*
- *2 teaspoons vanilla-infused jojoba oil (see page 92)*
- *8 drops Dry Skin Essential Oil Synergy (see page 51)*

5 MINUTES OR LESS

1 FLUID OUNCE, GOOD FOR 2 BODY SCRUB SESSIONS

Like the skin on your face, the skin on your body needs encouragement to shed dead skin cells and support for skin regeneration and rejuvenation. For those with ashy legs, scaly knees and elbows, and overall dry, flaky skin, this mild exfoliating scrub for dry skin offers a rich way to both slough away dead skin and nourish the new skin emerging below the surface. The star ingredient, almond meal, is rich in vitamin E, which not only heals skin but also acts as an effective antioxidant.

STEPS

1. In a small glass bowl, mix all the dry ingredients together and stir until well incorporated. Set aside.

2. Place the shea butter in another small glass bowl. If it feels lumpy, mash it down with the back of a stainless steel spoon until it is creamy. Then slowly drizzle the carrier oils into the shea butter with a whisk, stirring constantly until a light cream, with the consistency of yogurt, is formed.

3. At this point, pour the dry ingredients into the butter and oil blend, and mix well.

4. Add the synergy and stir until fully combined.

5. Scoop the final product into the glass jar and cap tightly. Store away from heat. The scrub should last for 2 weeks.

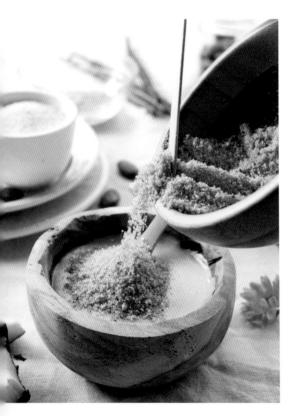
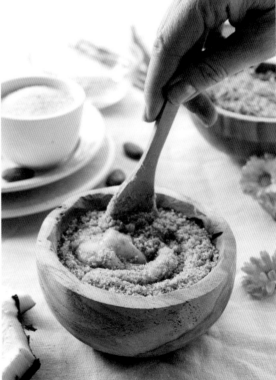

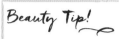

Beauty Tip!

How to Use the Body Scrub:

1. *Dampen your body, making sure to avoid sensitive areas.*
2. *Scoop out half the jar of body scrub and massage it in circular motions anywhere on your body that is in need of descaling and deep nourishment.*
3. *Apply more scrub if needed.*
4. *Rinse with a warm, wet washcloth.*

Beauty Note!

The sweet truth about using sugar for beauty: *Sugar, when applied topically, is a natural humectant, which means it attracts and absorbs water from the atmosphere to help skin absorb moisture. It is also full of glycolic acid, which loosens the gooey lipid mixture that holds the skin's cells together near the surface, so they can slough off more easily.[3] Sugar crystals can be softer on your skin than salt is, especially when moistened; they will leave your skin feeling softer and won't cause the microscopic tears that can sometimes occur when you use ground nuts or seeds. Also, since sugar softens when it comes in contact with warm water, providing a more soothing scrubby feeling, it is a better choice for more sensitive skin.*

Psst!

Make sure you use organic sugar (no one wants bleach residue on their skin) and avoid large-crystal sugar like Sugar in the Raw or other brands of turbinado sugar, as the larger crystals may scratch and irritate sensitive skin.

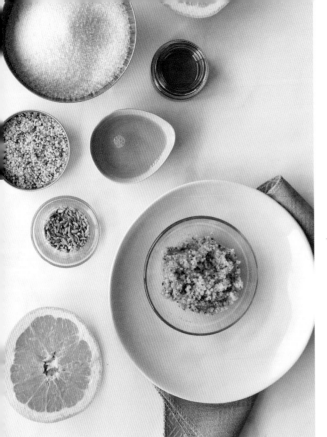

CELLULITE-BUSTER BODY SCRUB

- 2 small glass bowls
- 2 glass or wooden stirrers
- 1 (1-ounce) glass jar with a tight-fitting lid

- 1 tablespoon organic sugar
- 1 tablespoon ground hemp seeds
- 1 teaspoon unscented castile soap
- 1 teaspoon hemp seed oil
- 8 drops Cellulite-Buster Essential Oil Synergy (see page 51)

5 MINUTES OR LESS

1 FLUID OUNCE, GOOD FOR 1 OR 2 BODY SCRUB SESSIONS

Can we really get rid of cellulite? Probably not. But we can definitely improve the way it looks by increasing the health of our skin. Our suggestions include consistent exercise, mindful eating habits, and a strong skincare regimen that includes nutrient-rich, plant-based ingredients to release toxins and improve circulation.

STEPS

1. In a small glass bowl, stir together the sugar and hemp seeds until combined. Set aside.
2. In another small glass bowl, combine the castile soap and hemp seed oil, using a clean stirrer.
3. Pour the dry ingredients into the wet ingredients and mix well.
4. Add the synergy and mix until fully incorporated.

5. Scoop the finished product into the glass jar and cap tightly. Store in a dry location. The scrub should last for 1 month.

Beauty Note!

Hemp seeds are effective for reducing inflammation (puffiness), strengthening cellular membranes, promoting detoxification, fighting free radical damage, and evening out skin tone.[4] In this recipe, there is a double delivery of the supercharged components of this remarkable seed, (1) via the cold-pressed oil and (2) directly from the ground seeds, to ensure a potent dose of its anti-inflammatory and tissue-reparative properties.

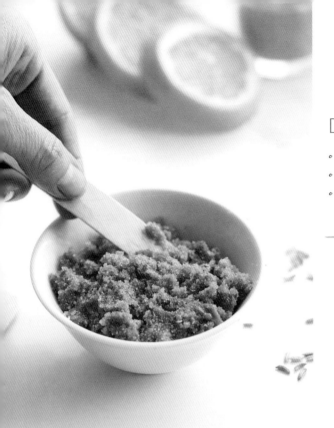

DETOX BODY SCRUB

- small glass bowl
- 2 glass or wooden stirrers
- 1 (1-ounce) glass jar with a tight-fitting lid

- 1 tablespoon finely ground Dead Sea salt
- 1 teaspoon fennel seed powder
- 1 teaspoon ginger powder
- 2 teaspoons sesame oil
- 8 drops Detox Body Essential Oil Synergy (see page 51)

5 MINUTES OR LESS

1 FLUID OUNCE, GOOD FOR 1 OR 2 BODY SCRUB SESSIONS

Our skin is a direct reflection of what is going on inside our bodies and how we react and respond to what happens externally. If we don't get enough sleep, or if we subsist on a diet heavy in fats, oils, and processed foods, our skin shows it. What can we do to help kick-start a healthier glow? A body scrub rich with ingredients known to improve circulation and release toxins from the body is a great way to start.

STEPS

1. In a small glass bowl, mix all the dry ingredients together and stir until combined.
2. Add the sesame oil and continue stirring.
3. Once the sesame oil and the dry ingredients are fully combined, add the synergy and mix to incorporate.
4. Scoop the mixture into the glass jar and cap tightly. Store in a dry location. The scrub should last for 2 months.

Beauty Note!

Salts in scrubs: Salt is effective at drawing out toxins, cleansing pores, and promoting healing. Interestingly, salt contains some of the same minerals and nutrients that exist in our own bodies, like calcium, magnesium, potassium, and sodium. So it makes sense that it can help us balance our own mineral content.

The salt we use in this recipe is from the Dead Sea in Israel, which yields salt with powerful healing effects on the skin due to its unique mineral content; this salt is able to draw out toxins and heal unrelenting wounds.[5] If finding Dead Sea salt proves challenging, you can substitute any kind of naturally mined salt, which will offer similar therapeutic properties. Some alternatives include Himalayan, French, or Celtic salt. Just make sure it is finely ground, so you don't risk making microscopic tears in the skin or breaking tiny capillaries.

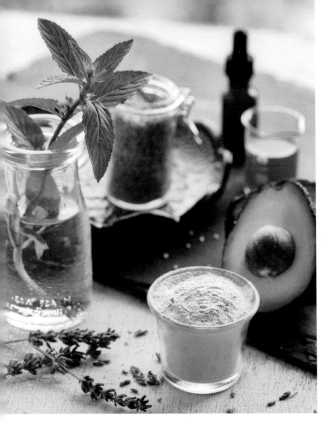

FOOT MASK

- small glass bowl
- glass or wooden stirrer
- 1 (2-ounce) glass jar with a tight-fitting lid

- 2 tablespoons bentonite clay powder
- 1 tablespoon dried lavender flower powder
- 20 drops Foot Mask Essential Oil Synergy (see page 51)

5 MINUTES OR LESS

2 FLUID OUNCES, GOOD FOR 1 OR 2 USES

Sometimes the best thing we can do for our feet is to get off them! And preparing and using a foot mask forces us to stop what we are doing and literally allow our feet to rest and rejuvenate. Our wonderful plant-powered foot mask is a great way to nourish and revive tired, achy feet and feed the skin of our soles.

Beauty Tip!

You will need about 1 tablespoon of additional wet ingredients— see the tip on the next page to activate the dry clay into a mask.

STEPS

1. In a small glass bowl, stir together the bentonite clay powder and dried lavender flower powder, making sure the clay and flower powders are well incorporated.
2. Add the synergy. You will notice small liquid droplets forming on the surface of the powders; use a stirrer to break them up and incorporate them into the powdered mixture until they are fully dissipated.
3. Transfer the blended ingredients to the glass jar, cap tightly, and give it a gentle shake. Store in a dry location. The mask should last for 3 months.

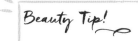

Beauty Tip!

How to Use the Foot Mask:

You will need 1½ teaspoons of avocado oil and 1½ teaspoons of sesame oil to activate the mask.

1. *In a small glass bowl, stir together the avocado oil and sesame oil.*
2. *Slowly, starting with 1 teaspoon, mix the dry clay powder blend with the oils until the consistency looks mud-like. If the mixture starts expanding and getting too thick, you can add more sesame oil or even a little water. Ideally you want the consistency to be soft and yogurt-like.*
3. *Wash your feet. Pat them down with a towel, leaving them a little damp. Or dry them completely and dampen with several spritzes of your favorite hydrosol to enhance the effect of the mask.*
4. *Using your fingers, smooth the mask all over the insides and outsides of your feet, making sure to get it between your toes.*
5. *Sit back and relax! The clay should start to harden in about 5 minutes. Allow yourself 5 to 10 minutes with the mask.*
6. *When the mask feels hardened and starts to crack a little, rinse your feet gently under warm water. Use a warm, wet washcloth to remove the residue.*

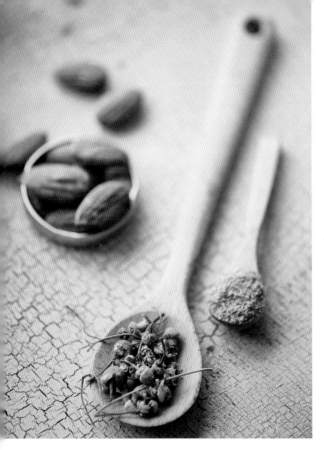

HAND MASK

- small glass bowl
- glass or wooden stirrer
- 1 (2-ounce) glass jar with a tight-fitting lid

- 2 tablespoons bentonite clay powder
- 1 teaspoon dried comfrey leaf powder
- 1 teaspoon dried chamomile flower powder
- 1 teaspoon organic raspberry fruit powder
- 15 drops Hand Mask Essential Oil Synergy (see page 51)

5 MINUTES OR LESS

2 FLUID OUNCES, GOOD FOR 1 OR 2 USES

As with our feet, we can easily forget about taking care of our hands. But coating our hands with a mask loaded with a botanical blast of rejuvenating ingredients can boost the way they look and feel. And the best part is that once the mask is on, we can't lift a finger!

Beauty Tip!

You will need about 1 tablespoon of additional wet ingredients—see opposire—to activate the dry clay into a mask.

STEPS

1. In a small glass bowl, combine all the dry ingredients, making sure all the powders are well incorporated.
2. Add the synergy. You will notice small liquid droplets forming on the surface of the powders; use a stirrer to break them up and incorporate them into the powdered mixture until they are fully dissipated.
3. Transfer the blended ingredients to the glass jar, cap tightly, and give it a gentle shake. Store in a dry location. The mask should last for 3 months.

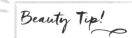

Beauty Tip!

How to Use the Hand Mask:

You will need 1 teaspoon of almond oil, 1 teaspoon of honey, and 1 teaspoon of vegetable glycerin to activate the mask.

1. *In a small glass bowl, stir together the almond oil, honey, and vegetable glycerin until well incorporated.*
2. *Slowly, starting with 1 teaspoon, mix the dry clay powder blend with the mixed wet ingredients until the consistency looks mud-like. If the mixture starts expanding and getting too thick, you can add more almond oil or a little water. Ideally you want the consistency to be soft and yogurt-like.*
3. *Lightly dampen your hands with warm water.*
4. *Using your fingers, smooth the mask all over the insides and outsides of your hands, making sure to get it between your fingers.*
5. *Sit back and relax! The clays should start to harden in about 5 minutes. Allow yourself 5 to 10 minutes with the mask.*
6. *When the mask feels hardened and starts to crack a little, rinse your hands gently under warm water. Use a warm, wet washcloth to remove the residue.*

Beauty Note!

Hydrosols for the hands: Try dampening your hands with a spritz of your favorite hydrosol before coating them with the mask. Dampening the skin before applying a mask or an oil treatment can help seal in added moisture, and with the added benefits of some of the plant molecules in hydrosols, you can give your hands a double treat. Any hydrosol will do the trick—just check out our nifty hydrosol chart on page 96.

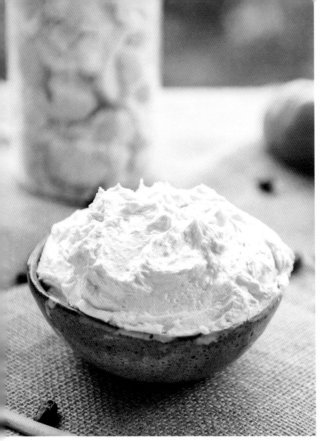

DREAMSICLE WHIPPED BODY BUTTER

- double boiler
- silicone spatula
- glass or wooden stirrer
- stand mixer or handheld mixer, with a whisk attachment
- 2 (8-ounce) glass jars with tight-fitting lids

- ¼ cup solid unrefined coconut oil
- ¼ cup refined or unrefined shea butter (see tips)
- ¼ cup cocoa butter (see tips)
- 4 tablespoons vanilla-infused jojoba oil (see page 92)
- 60 drops sweet orange essential oil

3 HOURS

16 OUNCES

Body butter is a rich moisturizer made without water. The omission of water simplifies the mixing procedure and there is less of a need to add a strong preservative system. Since all the ingredients are considered self-preserving, meaning on their own they have long shelf lives and very stable chemistries, we can opt for adding antioxidants, like vitamin E (tocopherol), without too much concern. Butters are our most nutrient-rich category of ingredients, providing a wide variety of healing properties for the skin.

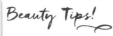

Beauty Tips!

Shea butter: *If you choose refined shea butter, make sure the process used is solvent-free.*
Cocoa butter: *Cocoa butter comes in both chips and large chunks. For this recipe, we like to use the un-deodorized and unrefined chips; they melt more easily, are easier to work with, and emit an intoxicating chocolate aroma.*

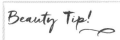

Beauty Tip!

Here are some fun variations for body butter formulating:

° *Replace half the cocoa butter with mango butter.*

° *Swap out the vanilla-infused jojoba oil with another herbal-infused oil, like calendula or comfrey, or replace the 4 tablespoons called for in the recipe with 1 tablespoon each of four different kinds of oils, like avocado, pumpkin seed, sesame, and almond.*

° *Use unrefined, un-deodorized coconut oil for a rich coconut scent.*

° *Create your own essential oil synergy using 3 to 5 essential oils, to boost the therapeutic actions of the butters and oils for deeper skin healing.*

STEPS

1. To set up the double boiler, pour 1½ inches of water into the bottom pot.

2. Add the coconut oil, shea butter, and cocoa butter directly into the top pot and melt slowly over very low heat.

3. Once all the butters are melted, stir to combine. Add the vanilla-infused jojoba oil, stir again, and turn off the heat.

4. Carefully lift the top pot of the double boiler (containing the melted butters and oils) off the bottom pot and dry the outside of the pot with a paper towel.

5. Pour the melted mixture into the glass or metal bowl you use with your stand or handheld mixer, and let the bowl cool for about 10 minutes.

6. Touch the side of the bowl to test the temperature. When it is no longer too hot to touch but still feels comfortably warm, transfer it to the refrigerator and place

a loose piece of parchment paper over it to prevent anything from dripping into it.

7. Let the bowl sit inside the fridge for about 1 to 2 hours, checking periodically. You will know the mixture is ready to whip when it has solidified and there is no gooey center.

8. Using the mixer's whisk attachment, whip the mixture on high for 3 minutes.

9. Pause the mixer and use a silicone spatula to scrape the mixture down from the sides of the bowl. Whip for another 1 to 2 minutes, until the butter starts to look like airy, fluffy frosting.

10. Scrape off as much butter as possible from the whisk attachment. If you are using a stand mixer, remove the bowl from the mixer.

11. Add the sweet orange essential oil and mix well using the spatula.

12. Transfer the body butter to the glass jars and cap tightly. Keep out of sunlight and away from heat. To prevent hardening, do not refrigerate. The body butter will last for 3 months.

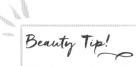

Beauty Tip!

The beauty benefits of body butters: *Why are butters such a great option for healing and nourishing the skin? Here are the top reasons why we love to use butters to moisturize our skin:*

- *They are rich in polyphenols, which protect against free radicals, oxidative stress, and UV rays.[6]*
- *They improve the flexibility of the skin.[7]*
- *They promote the regeneration of skin cells and the healing of wounds—they are great for softening scar tissue.*
- *They help skin retain moisture.*

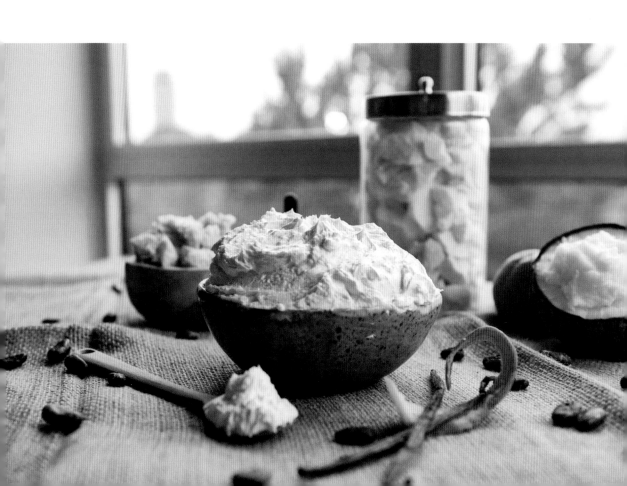

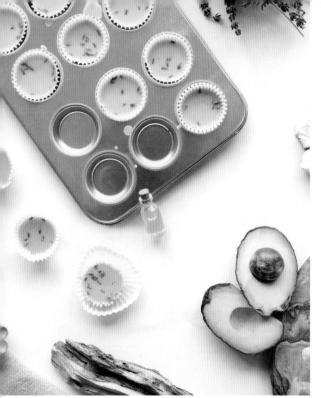

LOTION BARS

- ° *double boiler*
- ° *1 (8-ounce) glass measuring pitcher*
- ° *glass or wooden stirrer*
- ° *silicone candy or cupcake molds*

- ° *2 tablespoons beeswax pastilles*
- ° *2 tablespoons refined or unrefined shea butter (see tip)*
- ° *1 tablespoon solid unrefined coconut oil*
- ° *2 tablespoons avocado oil*
- ° *60 drops Dry Skin Essential Oil Synergy (see page 51)*

1 HOUR AND 15 MINUTES

THE YIELD OF THIS RECIPE REALLY DEPENDS ON THE SIZE OF YOUR MOLDS. WE MAKE THESE LOTION BARS WITH MINI CUPCAKE MOLDS, WHICH YIELD ABOUT 4 BARS.

Think of a lotion bar as a lip balm for the body. Shaped like a bar of soap, it is a handy skin soother, especially for really rough patches on knees, elbows, and feet. Once the lotion bar makes contact with the warmth of the skin, the oils and butters begin to melt and the skin is able to absorb many of the nutritious ingredients. Lotion bars are fun and unique delivery systems for moisturizing ingredients; they leave the skin feeling renewed without greasy residue.

STEPS

1. To set up the double boiler, pour about 1 inch of water into the bottom pot and about 1 inch of water into the upper pot. Turn the heat on medium to begin warming up the water in both the lower and upper pots.

2. Once the water begins to steam a bit, add the beeswax pastilles, shea butter, and coconut oil to a glass measuring pitcher and place it gently into the upper pot. Keep watch as the ingredients begin to melt. Stir occasionally.

Beauty Tip!

If you choose refined shea butter, make sure the process used is solvent-free.

3. Once the wax, shea butter, and coconut oil are fully melted and no remnants of the beeswax pastilles are visible, slowly pour in the avocado oil and stir to combine. Heat all the ingredients together and make sure everything is well incorporated.

4. Gently lift the warm measuring pitcher out of the top pot of the double boiler, and dry off the outside of the pitcher with a paper towel to prevent any drips of water from getting into the silicone molds.

5. Add the synergy and stir to combine.

6. Pour the warm melted mixture into the molds. Once the molds are filled, let the mixture cool on the counter for about 1 hour. We suggest covering the molds with parchment paper to prevent anything from dripping into them.

7. To remove lotion bars, gently push the bottom of the mold to individually pop them out.

Beauty Note!

Silicone molds are the very best to use. You can find them at any kitchen or home goods shop, and they come in a wide variety of shapes and sizes. If you use metal baking or candy molds, make sure you line the molds with parchment paper to help remove the lotion bars once they harden.

Try swapping out the avocado oil for a nut or seed oil, or an herbal-infused oil of your choice. We love avocado oil for its rich nutrient content and deep green color, which adds a pretty hue. But any nut or seed oil would work well. You could also try experimenting with the proportions and adding an extra 1 or 2 teaspoons of nut or seed oil to give the lotion bar a little more of a "melting factor" when it touches the skin.

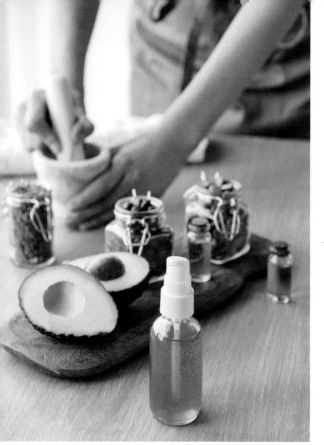

MOISTURIZING BODY OIL FOR SUPER-DRY SKIN

- glass bowl or beaker
- glass or wooden stirrer
- 1 (2-ounce) glass or non-BPA plastic bottle with a flip-top

- 4 teaspoons apricot kernel oil
- 4 teaspoons jojoba oil
- 4 teaspoons avocado oil
- 20 drops Dry Skin Essential Oil Synergy (see page 51)

10 MINUTES

2 FLUID OUNCES

Don't let the idea of using oil on your skin scare you away—plant-based nut and seed oils are nongreasy, nourishing, hydrating, and incredibly beneficial for your skin. They are infused with vitamins and help seal in moisture and humectants, preventing moisture from evaporating. As a bonus, the aroma released from the essential oil synergy we selected helps lift spirits for a complete mind-body pick-me-up.

STEPS

1. In a glass bowl or beaker, combine all the carrier oils and stir together.
2. Slowly add the synergy and stir to combine. The color of the blend should be pale green.
3. Transfer the mixture to the bottle, cap, and shake. It is now ready for use. Keep out of heat and away from

direct sunlight. To prevent hardening, do not refrigerate. The body oil should last for 4 months.

Beauty Tip!

How to Use Body Oil:

Body oils are best used when the skin is still damp, allowing for deeper penetration. We suggest applying daily when you get out of the shower or bath, after you lightly towel dry. A little oil goes a long way, so start with about 1 tablespoon in the palm of your hand and massage it into your skin where desired. Repeat for each section of your body, as needed.

BALANCING BODY OIL FOR SKIN HYDRATION AND MOOD BOOST

- *glass bowl or beaker*
- *glass or wooden stirrer*
- *1 (2-ounce) glass or non-BPA plastic bottle with a flip-top, dropper cap, or pump dispenser*

- *4 teaspoons sesame oil*
- *4 teaspoons apricot kernel oil*
- *4 teaspoons jojoba oil*
- *20 drops Balancing Essential Oil Synergy (see page 51)*

5 TO 10 MINUTES

2 FLUID OUNCES

Our skin can easily reflect our state of mind. Breakouts, rashes, irritations, or hives can be triggered by an emotional reaction or a psychological disposition. That's why we designed a body oil recipe to address both our mood and our skin simultaneously. This body oil can be an effective remedy when you are feeling overwhelmed and stressed.

STEPS

1. In a glass bowl or beaker, stir together all the carrier oils until fully incorporated. A rich golden color will emerge.

2. Add the synergy and keep stirring.

3. Transfer the mixture to the bottle, cap, and shake well for about 10 seconds. It is now ready for use. Keep in mind that over the next 24 hours or so the aroma will deepen and intensify. Keep out of heat and away from direct sunlight. To prevent hardening, do not refrigerate. The body oil should last for 4 months.

The Benefits of "Oiling" the Skin

Not all moisturizers are the same. There are creams and lotions and then there are body butters and oils. You might be wondering, what is the difference? And don't they all do the same things to our skin? Actually, there is a big difference. Skincare geeks like us actually have two categories: moisturizers and emollients.

Creams and lotions are generally classified as "moisturizers" because they are more complex formulations that include a whole range of ingredient categories that are designed specifically to help the skin attract and hold in water. You will also find that creams and lotions contain water as one of their main ingredients, while body oils do not. The water present in cream and lotion recipes is there solely to help deliver other ingredients to the skin; it is not included to hydrate or feed water to the skin. The skin can only be rehydrated when it is coated by a film that prevents water from evaporating from it.

Oils and butters are known as "emollients" (softeners) because they feed the "glue" that floats between our skin cells so that our skin maintains its smoothness, softness, elasticity, shape, and strength.[8] When this "glue" between the cells is well nourished, it prevents the skin from getting dehydrated and maintains the naturally occurring film that coats our skin.

So now that we understand the difference between creams and lotions and oils and butters, why would we reach for one over the other? Generally speaking, it has a lot to do with individual taste and how the product feels on our skin. Creams and lotions tend to be lighter, absorb more quickly, and may give the appearance of plumpness, whereas oils and butters tend to sit a little longer on the surface of the skin, may feel heavier and greasier, and give an appearance of shine and glow.

We usually suggest using oils and butters on skin that is extremely dry and damaged and needs some extra support to heal and regenerate. For example, they could be used for scars and healing wounds, scalp conditions, and wrinkle prevention.

Creams and lotions, on the other hand, are quite gentle for the face and perfect for areas of the body where we want to avoid a greasy look and feel. These kinds of emulsions are also recommended for skin that's been severely dehydrated and needs a quick-fix delivery of water before it receives nourishing fats.

Psst!

But which do we really prefer? Oiling up is definitely our favorite.

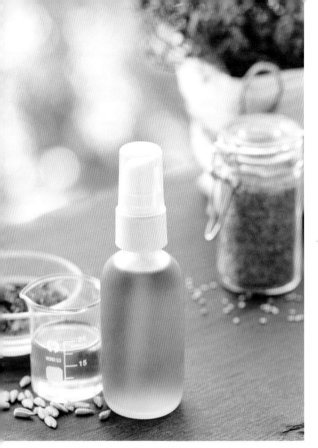

MASSAGE OIL FOR SORE MUSCLES

° *glass measuring pitcher*
° *glass or wooden stirrer*
° *1 (1-ounce) glass or non-BPA plastic bottle with a cap or dropper cap*

° *2 teaspoons sesame oil*
° *2 teaspoons sunflower seed oil*
° *1 teaspoon plantain-infused olive oil (see page 92)*
° *1 teaspoon comfrey-infused olive oil (see page 92)*
° *25 drops Sore Muscles Massage Oil Essential Oil Synergy (see page 52)*

5 MINUTES OR LESS

1 FLUID OUNCE, GOOD FOR 1 OR 2 FULL-BODY MASSAGE APPLICATIONS

Massage is a great way to ease away the discomfort of sore muscles. And applying a massage oil you blend yourself using essential oils and other plant-based components can improve circulation, relieve soreness, and lower stress.

STEPS

1. In a glass measuring pitcher, combine all the carrier oils and stir to incorporate.
2. Add the synergy and continue stirring.
3. Carefully transfer the mixture to the bottle, cap, and shake well. Keep out of heat and away from direct sunlight. To prevent hardening, do not refrigerate. The massage oil should last for 4 months.

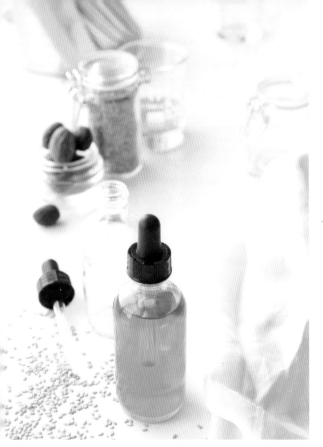

SEDUCTIVE MASSAGE OIL

° *glass bowl or beaker*
° *glass or wooden stirrer*
° *1 (1-ounce) glass bottle with a dropper*

° *1 tablespoon plus 1 teaspoon sesame oil*
° *2 teaspoons vanilla-infused jojoba oil (see page 92)*
° *25 drops Seductive Massage Essential Oil Synergy (see page 52)*

5 TO 10 MINUTES

1 FLUID OUNCE,

GOOD FOR 1 OR

2 FULL-BODY

MASSAGE

APPLICATIONS

The intoxicating aroma of the combined blend of ylang-ylang, patchouli, and nutmeg essential oils will stir your emotions, loosen your body, and awaken your heart.

STEPS

1. In a glass bowl or beaker, stir together the carrier oils.
2. Slowly add the synergy to the carrier oils and continue stirring for a few seconds until well incorporated.
3. Transfer the mixture to the glass bottle, cap, and shake. Keep out of heat and away from direct sunlight. To prevent hardening, do not refrigerate. The massage oil should last for 4 months.

Beauty Tip!

How to Use Massage Oil:

Pour 1 tablespoon of massage oil onto your hand, gently rub both hands together, and then apply to the desired area. Repeat for each area of the body.

Beauty Tip!

Rubbing and massaging the body with aromatic oils has been a practice for centuries. The benefits of massage include improving circulation; increasing mobility; relieving pain, soreness, and stiffness; and supporting lymphatic drainage. Massage can also be a very powerful psychological and emotional support by providing a touch connection between the giver and receiver. Even if you don't know anything about massage, a great way to begin is to gently place your hands on the area you want to massage and begin slow circular motions, increasing pressure and using your fingers to pulse, squeeze, and stroke the muscles. Sometimes just a soft pat can be incredibly soothing. Be attentive to how your partner reacts and incorporate their feedback.

Beauty Tip!

When making a massage blend, it is best to choose a carrier oil that will not absorb too quickly and will thus add a little slide to the touch. It is also a good idea to choose a selection of essential oils that can relax and ease muscle tightness.

PERSONAL CARE

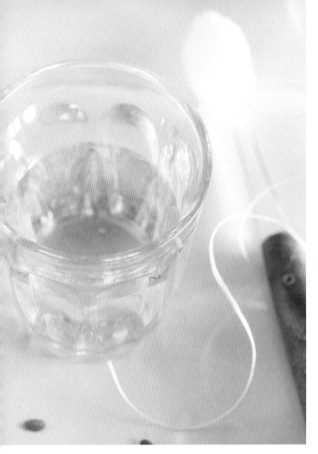

NATURAL MOUTHWASH

- glass or stainless steel bowl or glass beaker
- glass or wooden stirrer
- 1 (2-ounce) glass or non-BPA plastic bottle with a cap

- 1 drop peppermint essential oil
- 1 drop eucalyptus essential oil
- 1 drop cinnamon essential oil
- 1 drop marjoram essential oil
- 1 drop thyme essential oil
- 1 tablespoon vegetable glycerin
- 1 tablespoon distilled water
- 5 tablespoons lemon verbena hydrosol (see tip)

5 TO 10 MINUTES

2 FLUID OUNCES

Fresh breath does not have to rely on an over-the-counter mouthwash full of alcohol, sweeteners, and synthetic flavors. We use only plant-based ingredients to create a refreshing recipe bursting with authentic flavors and antiseptic and antimicrobial properties for a long-lasting clean mouth and fresh breath.

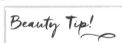

Beauty Tip!

You can substitute the lemon verbena hydrosol with peppermint, rosemary, lavender, or chamomile hydrosol

STEPS

1. In a bowl or beaker, stir together the five essential oils.
2. Add the vegetable glycerin and stir together.
3. Add the distilled water and lemon verbena hydrosol to the mixture and continue to stir.
4. Transfer the mixture to the bottle, cap, and shake. Keep out of heat and away from direct sunlight. To prevent hardening, do not refrigerate. The mouthwash should last for 2 months.

Beauty Tip!

You may notice that over time the essential oils rise to the top and form a golden halo. This is completely normal; simply shake before each use to fully reincorporate.

Beauty Tip!

How to Use Mouthwash: *After flossing and brushing your teeth, use about 1 tablespoon of mouthwash and swish generously around your mouth for about 30 seconds. Then spit out. Repeat as desired.*

Beauty Note!

Cinnamon essential oil: *A recent study by dental scientists in Chicago found that cinnamon essential oil effectively kills oral bacteria, including germs responsible for gum disease and bad breath.[1]*

Gum disease is caused by microorganisms in the mouth that damage and weaken our gums, sometimes no matter how diligent we are about brushing. Rinsing with a fully loaded combination of antimicrobials can help keep your gums fortified.[2]

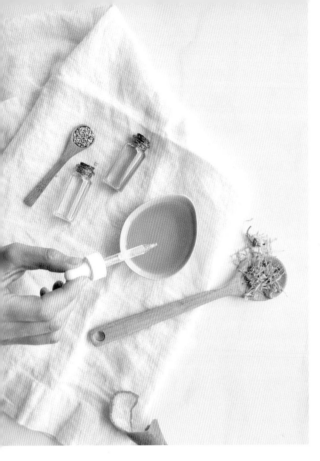

CUTICLE OIL

- *glass bowl or beaker*
- *glass or wooden stirrer*
- *1 (1-ounce) amber glass bottle with a dropper cap*

- *1 tablespoon sesame oil*
- *1½ teaspoons castor oil*
- *1½ teaspoons calendula-infused olive oil (see page 92)*
- *20 drops Cuticle Oil Essential Oil Synergy (see page 52)*

5 TO 10 MINUTES

1 FLUID OUNCE

Our cuticles are made up of dead skin cells and serve a key function—protecting the seal of the back of the visible nail with a barrier that keeps bacteria out and prevents infection. When cuticles are dry and brittle, they are not as effective in their protective role. Therefore, regular moisturizing is essential for nail health and beautification. Our cuticle oil is simple to make and is a recommended addition to your arsenal of beauty supplies for daily use.

STEPS

1. In a glass bowl or beaker, combine all the carrier oils and stir together.
2. Add the synergy and continue stirring until fully combined.
3. Transfer the mixture to the glass bottle, cap, and shake

well. Keep out of heat and away from direct sunlight. To prevent hardening, do not refrigerate. The cuticle oil should last for 4 months.

Beauty Tip!

How to Use Cuticle Oil:

Apply 1 drop of oil to each cuticle and gently massage in. Repeat twice daily or as desired.

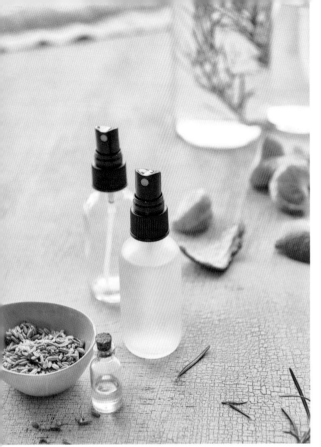

NATURAL SPRAY DEODORANT

- 2 glass or stainless steel bowls or glass beakers
- small stainless steel whisk
- 1 (2-ounce) glass or non-BPA plastic bottle with a spray top

- 1 teaspoon vegetable glycerin
- 25 drops Detox Essential Oil Synergy (see page 51)
- 1 tablespoon rosemary hydrosol (see tip)
- 5 teaspoons witch hazel

5 TO 10 MINUTES

2 FLUID OUNCES

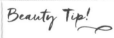

Beauty Tip!

Rosemary hydrosol can be replaced with other hydrosols such as lavender, Douglas fir, lemon verbena, melissa, or rose geranium. Try a hydrosol that has known antimicrobial actions.

Conventional antiperspirants and deodorants often contain concerning ingredients like aluminum,[3] parabens,[4] and triclosan.[5] And there has been mounting research suggesting it's probably best to limit their usage. An alternative? Our Natural Spray Deodorant, made with ingredients like witch hazel (a natural antimicrobial and astringent) and rosemary hydrosol, offers antifungal properties and a fresh, clean scent.

STEPS

1. In a bowl or beaker, combine the vegetable glycerin and synergy.
2. In a separate bowl or beaker, mix the rosemary hydrosol and witch hazel.
3. Once they are well combined, slowly drizzle the hydrosol and witch hazel mixture into the first bowl containing

the vegetable glycerin and essential oil blend, continually whisking to completely incorporate all ingredients.

4. Transfer the blend to the bottle. Affix the top and shake to further combine the ingredients. Keep out of heat and away from direct sunlight. To prevent hardening, do not refrigerate. The deodorant should last for 4 months.

Beauty Tip!

How to Use Natural Spray Deodorant:

1. Make sure your skin is completely clean.
2. Point the nozzle of your deodorant bottle at the body part you wish to spray and hold the bottle several inches away. Spray once or twice, as desired, and reapply when necessary.

Beauty Note!

What's the difference between a deodorant and an antiperspirant? Deodorants neutralize odors triggered by the reaction between our sweat and the microorganisms living on our skin, while antiperspirants inhibit the excretion of our sweat glands. When formulated correctly using plant-based antimicrobial molecules, deodorants can have a significant effect in balancing out the ecosystem of our skin's microflora and reducing unpleasant odors.

PAIN RELIEF GEL

- glass measuring pitcher
- glass or wooden stirrer
- 1 (1-ounce) non-BPA plastic bottle with a squeeze top dispenser

---

- *25 drops Pain Relief Gel Essential Oil Synergy (see page 53)*
- *1 tablespoon plus 1 teaspoon aloe vera gel (make sure to use "gel" and not "juice")*
- *1 teaspoon lavender hydrosol*

5 TO 10 MINUTES

1 FLUID OUNCE

We blended essential oils famous for their pain-relieving qualities with the soothing action of aloe vera and lavender hydrosol to craft a nontoxic pain relief gel that goes right to work on sore muscles.

Beauty Tip!

How to Use Pain Relief Gel:

Squeeze out a nickel-size portion of the gel onto the palm of your hand and massage into the affected area. Use as often as needed.

STEPS

1. In a glass measuring pitcher, combine all the ingredients. Mix together to fully incorporate.
2. Transfer the mixture to the plastic bottle and close tightly. Keep refrigerated to activate the cooling, anti-inflammatory properties. The gel should last for 1 month.

Beauty Note!

We love working with aloe vera gel because of its fast penetrating action and amazing ability to reduce inflammation—important features for managing pain relief. Its soothing and cooling texture and light feel on the skin also make aloe vera gel less messy and more usable than some other products during a busy day.

Know Your Pain Relief Essential Oils

Sweet birch is a specialty essential oil (exuding a wintergreen aroma) that has been used as a pain reliever throughout history. *Warning*: Birch should not be used by anyone allergic to aspirin or currently on blood thinner medication, and should *never* be taken orally. We also strongly recommend that this essential oil never be used on children under the age of fifteen, the elderly, pregnant women, or anyone with a compromised immune system.

Marjoram is an herbaceous, oregano-like scented oil that is steam-distilled from the leaves of the marjoram herb, the same plant we use for cooking. Prized for its strong antispasmodic actions and warming effect, marjoram offers soothing relief for over-worked, stressed, or achy muscles.

Peppermint is a bright and uplifting essential oil that delivers powerful pain relief. It is regularly used for muscle, joint, and nerve pain, as well as headaches. The refreshing smell comes from a particular molecule called menthol. Peppermint essential oil is very irritating to the skin, especially to mucus membranes, so make sure it never touches your skin directly and keep it away from your face. If by accident you get a little on a sensitive area, use some of our Coconut Whip Makeup Remover (see page 190) to wipe it away. Like sweet birch, this oil should not be used on children.

Lavender has a wide array of aromatic components that make it smell both camphor-like and sweetly minty, as well as floral, fresh, and grassy. It has a strong sedative effect and possesses anti-inflammatory and analgesic properties that are wonderful for addressing sore muscles.

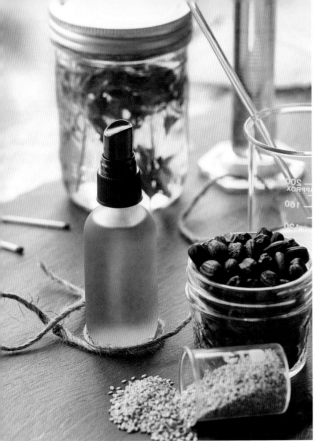

OIL-BASED BUG SPRAY FOR THE BODY

- glass measuring pitcher
- glass or wooden stirrer
- 1 (1-ounce) glass or non-BPA plastic bottle with a fine mist sprayer

- 1 tablespoon sesame oil
- 1 tablespoon jojoba oil
- 20 drops Bug Spray Essential Oil Synergy (see page 53)

5 MINUTES OR LESS

1 FLUID OUNCE, GOOD FOR 1 OR 2 FULL-BODY APPLICATIONS

Plant-based oils, especially vegetable oils combined with essential oils, can be tremendously effective against insects. After all, the reason the plant manufactures essential oils is to actually attract or ward off insects. Since we understand that our skin absorbs much of what is put on it, there is a growing concern about the high levels of potentially harmful and irritating chemical compounds that are present in many over-the-counter bug repellents. Mindful of this concern, we came up with a natural blend that has been tried and tested in many buggy environments.

STEPS

1. In a glass measuring pitcher, mix the sesame oil and jojoba oil together.
2. Add the synergy and stir until combined.
3. Slowly transfer the mixture to the spray bottle, cap, and

Beauty Tip!

A glass bottle is preferred, but plastic is advised for travel to avoid breakage.

shake well. Keep out of heat and away from direct sun-light. To prevent hardening, do not refrigerate. The bug spray should last for 4 months.

Beauty Tip!

Why did we choose jojoba oil and sesame seed oil for our bug spray? Two reasons:

1. *Jojoba oil absorbs quickly into the skin and doesn't leave a greasy feel, so it won't make your skin feel wet and hot if you are working or playing outside. Plus, since chemically it resembles more of a liquid wax than a vegetable oil, it won't go rancid in the heat.*
2. *Sesame oil has many antimicrobial properties, which is an added plus when trying to ward off insects.*

Combined together, the two oils lightly coat the skin and provide a nongreasy protective barrier, while safely dispersing the strong combi-nation of the Bug Spray Essential Oil Synergy.

WATER-BASED BUG SPRAY FOR CLOTHES

- glass measuring pitcher
- glass or wooden stirrer
- 1 (1-ounce) glass or non-BPA plastic bottle with a fine mist sprayer

---

- 1 teaspoon organic high-proof alcohol (such as Everclear grain alcohol, though any brand of vodka will work)
- 20 drops Bug Spray Essential Oil Synergy (see page 53)
- 2 tablespoons distilled water

5 MINUTES OR LESS

1 FLUID OUNCE, GOOD FOR 1 OR 2 FULL-BODY APPLICATIONS

This safe, nonstaining bug spray blend can be applied directly to clothes to ward off insects. The essential oil synergy is the same as the one in the Oil-Based Bug Spray for the Body, but we have switched up the delivery so it can be easily sprayed on socks, pants, shirts, and hats when you venture outside into bug-laden territory.

STEPS

1. In a glass measuring pitcher, combine the alcohol and synergy. Mix well until the essential oils look like they are no longer separating from the alcohol.
2. Once the mixture is fully blended, add the distilled water and mix well.
3. Transfer the mixture to the spray bottle, cap, and shake vigorously. Keep out of heat and away from direct sunlight. To prevent hardening, do not refrigerate. The bug spray should last for 4 months.

Beauty Tip!

A glass bottle is preferred, but plastic is advised for travel to avoid breakage.

Beauty Note!

Alcohol and essential oils: *Alcohol helps solubilize essential oils into water for beauty blending. The trick is to use a high proof in a small quantity. Since essential oils are hydrophobic, meaning they can't dissolve in water on their own, they need an "agent" to help them break down. Without alcohol, the essential oils will separate and float on the top, and there is a risk that microscopic droplets of pure essential oils may get on the skin and cause irritation. In this recipe, the essential oils included to create an effective bug repellent are known to be very irritating to the skin, so we added a little alcohol to avoid any chance of irritation.*

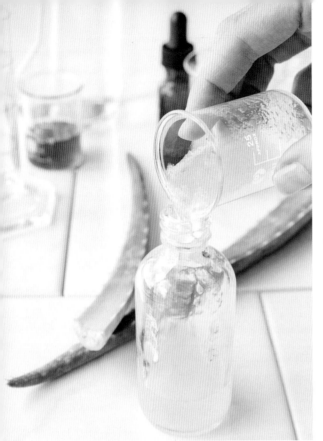

HEALTHY HAND-SANITIZING GEL

- small glass bowl
- glass or wooden stirrer
- 1 (2-ounce) plastic bottle with a flip-top

- *3 tablespoons aloe vera gel (look for inner fillet type)*
- *1 tablespoon witch hazel*
- *2 drops vitamin E*
- *20 drops Healthy Hand-Sanitizing Essential Oil Synergy (see page 53)*

5 MINUTES OR LESS

2 FLUID OUNCES

Washing our hands with natural soap and warm water is the ideal way to reduce germs in many situations.[6] However, when we are on the go, using a hand sanitizer can be the next best thing. Our healthy hand sanitizer recipe is made with essential oils containing antimicrobial and antifungal properties, along with aloe vera to keep hands soft and smooth. In contrast to the many alcohol-based blends on the market that dry skin out, our hand-sanitizing gel works to moisturize while keeping your hands germ-free.

STEPS

1. In a small glass bowl, combine the aloe vera gel and witch hazel and stir until fully incorporated.
2. Add the vitamin E followed by the synergy and continue stirring until the ingredients are fully combined.

3.   Transfer the formula to the plastic bottle, close the bottle, and shake. Keep out of heat and away from direct sunlight. The gel should last for 2 months.

Beauty Tip!

Add 1 or 2 drops of lemon essential oil for an extra citrus zing and a formidable detoxifying dose of antiseptic and immune-enhancing powers. In addition to these impressive properties, lemon essential oil is known to lift emotions—what a great bonus to having clean hands!

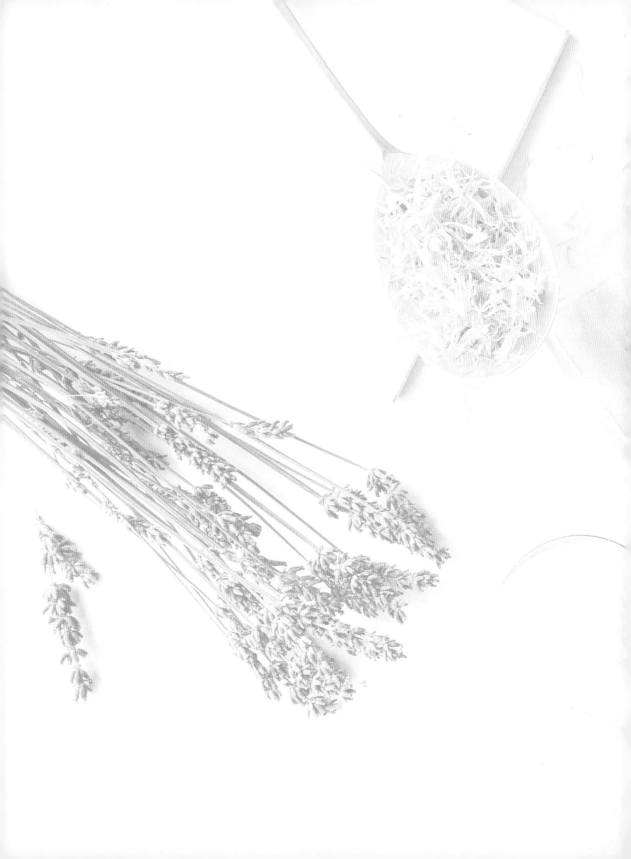

MIND-BODY CARE

NOURISHING AROMATHERAPY BATH TEA BAG

- glass or stainless steel bowl
- 1 large reusable or disposable tea bag (see tip)

- 4 tablespoons Dead Sea salt
- 1 tablespoon dried calendula flowers
- 1 tablespoon dried lavender flowers
- 2 teaspoons matcha powder
- 6 drops Sensitive Skin Essential Oil Synergy (see page 51)

5 TO 10 MINUTES

1 BATH TEA BAG

Aromatherapy tea bags for the bath offer a beautiful way to sooth nerves and soften skin while enjoying the fragrant and healing power of essential oils, dried flowers, and herbs. They also make beautiful gifts, so there is always an excuse to have your bouquet of ingredients on hand.

Beauty Tip!

Reusable tea bags are made of cotton muslin and have little drawstrings to tie them shut. Disposable tea bags look like little coffee filters that you can fold or tuck shut. You should find a size about 2½ inches wide and 4 inches long.

STEPS

1. In a glass or stainless steel bowl, stir together all the dry ingredients.
2. Gently add the synergy and stir together, allowing the essential oils to fold into the dry ingredients. Allow the mixture to sit for about 20 seconds.
3. Transfer all the ingredients to a tea bag. You can use the bath tea bag immediately or label it and store it in an airtight container for later use (or to give as a gift!). If properly stored, bath tea bags can last for 2 months.

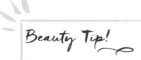

Beauty Tip!

How to Use the Bath Tea Bag:

1. Start by filling your tub with water for your bath.
2. Fill a bowl with a few cups of boiled water, then add your tea bag and let it steep for about 10 minutes. By doing this, you are truly making tea for your bath!
3. Pour the entire bowl of tea along with the tea bag into your bath.
4. Check the temperature of the water and adjust as needed. Then slip into your tub and soak for 20 minutes, enjoying the aroma and skin-loving effects of the tea-infused bathwater.

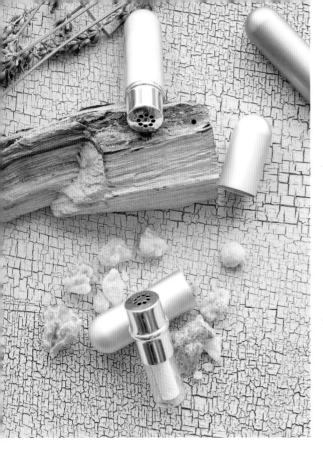

INHALER FOR CALMING/SOOTHING

 ° **25 drops Calming/Soothing Essential Oil Synergy (see page 53)**

INHALER FOR MOOD LIFTING

 ° **25 drops Mood-Lifting Essential Oil Synergy (see page 53)**

Inhalers offer a convenient way to transport essential oils in a pocket-size device (about the shape and size of a lip balm) so you can have them ready anytime. When you smell an essential oil or synergy, the aroma molecules send signals to the limbic system—the area of the brain that manages emotions, also known as the "emotional brain." This can spark positive feelings and, depending on the essential oils selected, help address a host of problems like anxiety, insomnia, and nervousness, to name just a few.

- small glass or stainless steel bowl
- glass or wooden stirrer
- 1 inhaler container with a cotton swab

STEPS

1. Add the synergy to a small glass or stainless steel bowl.
2. Take the cotton swab insert that comes with the inhaler and drop it into the pool of essential oils, letting it soak up the oils for several minutes. To help ensure a full soaking, you may wish to move the cotton swab around with a glass or wooden stirrer.
3. Once the oils are completely soaked into the cotton swab, remove it from the bowl using a stirrer and place it into the inhaler tube.
4. Close the tube by twisting the closure in place firmly and then place the cap on. Presto! You now have an inhaler ready to use. An essential oil inhaler lasts about 1 week before the aroma begins to fade away, so be sure to use it when it is fresh.

5 TO 10 MINUTES

1 INHALER

Beauty Tip!

How to Use the Inhaler:

To use the inhaler, simply remove the cap, hold the device up to one nostril, gently close the other nostril, and inhale. You can use the inhaler several times a day or as needed.

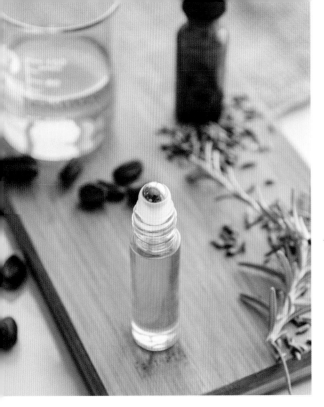

ROLL-ON FOR ACHY HEADS

- glass measuring pitcher
- glass or wooden stirrer
- 1 (0.35-ounce) glass roll-on bottle with a cap

- 2¼ teaspoons jojoba oil
- 36 drops Roll-On for Headaches Essential Oil Synergy (see page 53)

5 MINUTES OR LESS

1 (0.35-OUNCE) ROLL-ON

Headaches can be caused by many different reasons, like allergies, cold and flu, hormones, stress, and tension, but they can share identical symptoms. This recipe focuses solely on soothing the discomfort so we can feel better.

STEPS

1. In a glass measuring pitcher, combine the jojoba oil and synergy, mixing well.

2. Carefully pour the mixture into the narrow opening of the roll-on bottle. Snap the roller ball into place, cap the bottle, and shake. The roll-on should last for 6 months.

Beauty Tip!

How to Use the Roll-On:

Gently roll the oil blend on your temples, the back of your neck, and your scalp. Use as often as needed when symptoms arise.

ROLL-ON FOR CALMING/SOOTHING

- *2 teaspoons jojoba oil*
- *36 drops Calming/Soothing Essential Oil Synergy (see page 53)*

ROLL-ON FOR MOOD LIFTING

- *2 teaspoons jojoba oil*
- *36 drops Mood-Lifting Essential Oil Synergy (see page 53)*

In all our roll-on recipes we use jojoba oil as the base ingredient because it has a stable shelf life and helps "carry" the essential oil benefits into the skin. Roll-ons are safe for all skin types and they provide many therapeutic benefits. So whether you are looking for a mood boost, an aid for relaxation, or a remedy for sore muscles, roll-ons are a simple and compact solution.

- *1 (0.35-ounce) glass roll-on bottle with a cap*

5 MINUTES OR LESS

1 (0.35-OUNCE) ROLL-ON

STEPS

1. Add the synergy to the roll-on bottle.
2. Add the jojoba oil to the roll-on bottle.
3. Snap the roller ball into place, cap the bottle, and shake to combine the oils. The roll-on is now ready for use. The roll-on should last for 6 months.

Beauty Tip!

How to Use the Roll-On:

Shake before each use, then remove the cap and apply the roller ball to pressure points on your body, such as your wrists, your temples, the bottoms of your feet, or anywhere that feels good.

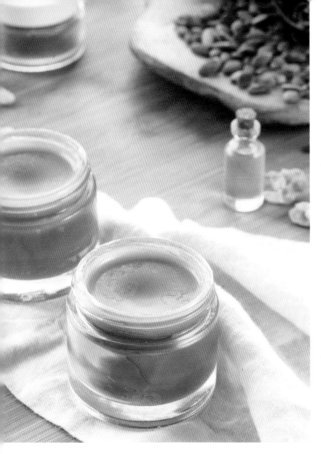

SALVE FOR MINDFULNESS

- 1½ teaspoons organic unrefined beeswax pastilles
- 2 tablespoons baobab seed oil
- 2 tablespoons pumpkin seed oil
- 30 drops Calming/Soothing Essential Oil Synergy (see page 53)

SALVE FOR BALANCING

- 1½ teaspoons beeswax pastilles
- 2 tablespoons calendula-infused herbal oil (see page 92)
- 1 tablespoon hemp seed oil
- 1 tablespoon jojoba oil
- 30 drops Balancing Essential Oil Synergy (see page 51)

A salve is a blend of wax (such as beeswax or candelilla wax) and carrier oils (like sunflower or apricot kernel) that when melted and mixed together create an oil-like cream or ointment. Salves have traditionally been used by herbalists to heal wounds, soften scars, soothe troubled skin, and support both breathing and digestion. By experimenting with slight variations in the ratio of wax to oil, you can customize your salve to be either more ointment-like or more solid in consistency.

Beauty Tip!

How to Use the Salve:

Scoop one fingerful of the salve into the palm of your hand and dab on your temples, neck, and upper chest. Use as often as needed.

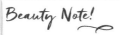

Beauty Note!

Baobab ingredient spotlight: *The baobab tree is originally from Africa and is often referred to as the Tree of Life because it provides both shelter and sustenance. In fact, every part of the tree—its cork bark, trunk, leaves, and fruit—shelters and feeds both humans and animals. It symbolizes a deep soulful nourishment, reminding us to be more peaceful.*

Balms versus salves: *Many people are confused about the difference between balms and salves, and some even mistake them for the same thing. Just remember that a balm is made with butters and beeswax, while a salve is made with simply beeswax and oil.*

- *double boiler*
- *2 glass measuring pitchers*
- *glass or wooden stirrer*
- *1 (1-ounce) glass jar with a tight-fitting lid*

2 HOURS AND

15 MINUTES

1 FLUID OUNCE

STEPS

1. To set up the double boiler, pour about 1 inch of water into the bottom pot and about 1 inch of water into the upper pot. Turn the heat on medium to begin warming up the water in both the lower and upper pots.

2. Once the water begins to steam a bit, add the beeswax pastilles to the first glass measuring pitcher and place it gently into the upper pot. Keep watch as the beeswax pastilles begin to melt.

3. While the beeswax is heating up, add the carrier oils to the second glass measuring pitcher. Stir to mix the oils together.

4. Once the beeswax is fully melted and no remnants of the pastilles are visible, slowly pour in the blended oils, and mix together.

5. The melted beeswax may harden a little when the oils are poured in. If that happens, don't worry; simply use a glass or wooden stick to stir the mixture as it is heating to make sure the beeswax remelts and the oils incorporate completely.

6. While the mixture is heating, add the synergy to the glass storage jar.

7. Carefully lift the warm measuring pitcher out of the top pot of the double boiler, and dry off the outside of the pitcher with a paper towel to prevent any drips of water from getting into the jar.

8. Pour the warm melted salve into the jar containing the synergy and cap it tightly.

9. Let the jar set without shaking or mixing the contents, until the salve hardens and cools. This could take about 2 hours. Keep out of heat and away from direct sunlight. The salve should last for 6 months.

Beauty Tip!

If you want the texture and consistency of your salve to always be the same every time you make it, it is important to measure the waxes and butters by dry weight, rather than fluid ounces. This way you can replicate the recipe exactly and use more precision in determining your customized ratios of oil to wax.

Beauty Tip!

Ingredients for mind-body balancing: *We turn to herbal-infused oils strong in anti-inflammatory actions when seeking to bring the body and mind back into balance. It is not only our skin and muscles that get inflamed but also our moods. And herbal-infused oils, like calendula, which is used in this recipe, have been shown to soothe wounds and reduce inflammation. When we combine them with seed oils rich in essential fatty acids, like hemp seed, we produce a remedy for both physical and emotional balancing.*

CBD CARE

CBD Care

Recipes

CBD is everywhere, right? We see it listed as an ingredient in everything, including toothpastes, pain creams, face oils, scalp treatments, and even deodorants. So what is it, and why is everyone excited about using it?

CBD, or cannabidiol, is a unique molecule that exists within the *Cannabis sativa* plant, also known by its common names, hemp and marijuana. CBD is the second-most-abundant cannabinoid found in the cannabis plant, following THC, or tetrahydrocannabinol. Cannabinoids are compounds found only in hemp and marijuana. What differentiates hemp and marijuana is variation in their cannabinoid composition: "industrial hemp" has less than 0.3 percent THC, and marijuana has more than 0.3 percent THC. Both (usually) have a rich quantity of CBD. Note: THC is psychoactive. CBD is *not* psychoactive.

Before we launch into details about CBD, let's step back for a moment and talk about plants and plant medicine. All plants are composed of hundreds of different phytochemical molecules and compounds. And these molecules give plants their identifying characteristics and medicinal and therapeutic properties. For example, the aroma we recognize as mint is actually one particular molecule that is part of the complex phytochemical composition of the peppermint plant. Another example is chamomile. We all have experienced how soothing chamomile tea can be. This soothing action is triggered by specific chemical compounds that are an integral part of the chamomile plant's flowers and leaves and are drawn out of the plant material by the warm water when we make tea.

The key to the practice of herbal medicine is understanding that all plants are composed of a wide variety of different phytochemicals. Depending on how we extract these different components and then use those extractions, the molecules in the extractions, when ingested or applied topically, can deeply affect our physiology and mental state.

This is all to say that CBD is a phytochemical that offers its very own unique set of therapeutic properties—especially when teamed up with other cannabinoids and plant compounds.

Research has shown that CBD has a powerful effect on our physiology, from reducing pain and inflammation to promoting tissue repair, fortifying our immunity, soothing our nervous system, and supporting our endocrine system.

Endocannabinoid System

As researchers have studied *why* the CBD molecule has such a powerful effect on our physiology, they have learned about the dynamic, complex, and elegant web of neurons and cells that compose our endocannabinoid system (ECS).

What exactly is the endocannabinoid system?

The human body is an astonishing machine that is constantly in motion—navigating our environment, supporting our growth, healing our tissues, protecting us—and all that is ultimately masterminded by our endocannabinoid system. The ECS's main role is to help maintain balance amid the constant barrage of stressors that bombard us. This amazing network of cells is constantly communicating with our immune system, our endocrine system, and our nervous system to make sure we stay healthy and balanced.

But what happens if the ECS can't keep everything in sync? The result is that we don't feel well and we start feeling the symptoms of imbalance, like inflammation, anxiety, and pain.

So imagine if we could apply or ingest something that could help our ECS get back into balance . . .

That something is CBD.

CBD communicates with the cells of our ECS and helps that system find its way back to balance. When our body is cruising in that state of balance, our immune system is better fortified against threats, and we are more likely to be able to fight off sickness and even disease.

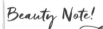

Beauty Note!

This might be a good place to revisit the skin anatomy chapter (page 31) to brush up on the structure and function of our skin

How does this relate to the health and appearance of our skin? The ECS is present in every organ of our bodies, including our skin. That means that if we are experiencing symptoms like itching, acne breakouts, or just simple signs of aging, our ECS may not be working as effectively and efficiently as it could. In this chapter, you'll learn about several CBD-infused recipes for health and wellness that can help restore balance to our ECS.

CBD Extractions

As you embark on blending your own CBD products, it is important to understand the different types of CBD extractions and methods so you can select CBD oil that meets your therapeutic goals and blending principles. We consulted with our friend and colleague Mia Davis, a clean beauty pioneer and hemp oil expert, on what to look for. Mia says, "Start with hemp that has been grown organically in the United States. Your supplier should have no problem tracing the oil you're buying right back to the hemp plant it came from—and they should share that information with you. In addition, they should be happy to disclose their extraction methods and the test results of the finished oil that break down the amounts of CBD, THC, and other major cannabinoids, as well as the results of pesticide and heavy metal testing." She also provides the descriptions in the chart on page 273—thanks, Mia!

CBD EXTRACTION

Type of CBD Extraction	Description
Full-Spectrum Extract	*The plant oil is extracted from the whole hemp plant. In this process, CBD is present along with other cannabinoids and therapeutic compounds such as terpenes, amino acids, vitamins, and minerals. Less than 0.3 percent of THC is present.*
Broad-Spectrum Extract	*CBD and other compounds found within the plant are present. THC is completely removed.*
Isolate	*In this process, a chemical compound is isolated and pulled out of the plant. It is pure and solitary.*

Extraction Method	Description
Lipid	*This ultra-natural process utilizes the whole plant and a fat (such as coconut oil). This oil is full spectrum and involves no manipulation or processing. The drawback is that the oil is green, smelly, and more likely to go "off."*
CO_2	*CO_2 is pressurized in metal tanks until it becomes a supercritical fluid; then the fluids pull out the desirable compounds from the flower. This is a very clean method, using no solvents.*
Ethanol Extraction	*Raw cannabis is soaked in ethanol; then the cannabis is removed and the liquid and alcohol are filtered from the extracted plant material. Ethanol is generally recognized as a safe ingredient, and none of it is left in the finished oil.*
Hydrocarbon	*Propane or butane is passed through raw cannabis as a solvent to collect cannabinoids and terpenes. Then the solvent with the essential oils is heated up to remove the propane or butane, leaving behind the extract.*

Figuring Out the Potency of Your CBD Extract

Before you experiment with CBD in your plant-powered skincare products, you need to know (1) the extraction method, (2) the quality of the extraction, and (3) the number of milligrams of CBD in the ingredient you purchased.

The amounts of CBD we provide in our recipes are based on specs from Hudson Hemp, where we purchase our distillate. Not all suppliers will have the same ratio of CBD per teaspoon, so be aware that your teaspoon of distillate may not equal the same amount of milligram of CBD as ours. Chances are that your CBD supplier has diluted the extract into an oil, like MCT oil, olive oil, or hempseed oil (remember, CBD isn't soluble in water). Make sure you ask which oil is used if you aren't sure.

Beauty Note!

These measurements are approximate. Since oils have different weights, one drop of one oil may be heavier or lighter than another.

Most important, you need to find out how many milligrams of CBD has been dissolved into the oil. For example, let's say you purchased a 10 ml bottle of CBD from a supplier and they tell you that the bottle contains 250 grams of CBD. That means every milliliter contains 25 grams of CBD.

OIL MEASUREMENTS

Drops	Teaspoon (tsp)	Milliliter (ml)
20	.20	1
40	.40	2
60	.60	3
80	.80	4
100	1	5

3 teaspoons = 1 tablespoon
2 tablespoons = 1 ounce

How Much CBD Is Needed to Be Effective?

The research on this is still not conclusive, and how much we absorb through the skin is entirely dependent on a wide array of factors like pore size, skin temperature, friction, type of product, where the product is applied, and so on. So, whether you use CBD sparingly or slather it on, the effect is generally anecdotal—meaning we recommend that you experiment and observe, take good notes, and see how much you need to feel and see an effect. But from our experience, we suggest starting with at least 150 milligrams or more per ounce of product.

The Entourage Effect

A great way to enhance the effect of CBD on our bodies and minds is by blending it with essential oils. Essential oils are made up of chemical compounds classified as *terpenes*, and this unique class of chemical components works synergistically with cannabidiol, which is from a different class of chemical compounds called *cannabinoids*. Even though essential oils and cannabidiol are from different classes of chemical compounds, they resonate well with each other since they mostly make up the volatile and aromatic parts of the plants' chemistry. This unique relationship between a few key essential oils and CBD is part of what is called the *entourage effect*.

See the chart on the next page for a few key essential oils that have been shown to enhance the therapeutic effects of CBD.

	METHOD OF EXTRACTION	SAFETY CONCERNS
BLACK PEPPER /PIPER NIGRUM		
PARTS USED: *dried fruit* **PRICE POINT:** *medium to high* **CAN SUBSTITUTE FOR/WITH:** *ginger, cardamom*	*steam distillation*	*avoid direct application to skin,* *avoid if pregnant, always dilute*
COPAIBA /COPAIFERA OFFICINALIS		
PARTS USED: *resin* **PRICE POINT:** *medium* **CAN SUBSTITUTE FOR/** **WITH:** *frankincense, myrrh,* *sandalwood, Atlas cedarwood*	*steam distillation*	*none*
JUNIPER /SEE ESSENTIAL OIL CHART ON PAGES 58–59.		
LAVENDER /SEE ESSENTIAL OIL CHART ON PAGES 58–59.		
LEMON /SEE ESSENTIAL OIL CHART ON PAGES 60–61.		

Regulations

The CBD regulatory landscape is constantly evolving. As we write this book, CBD (and other cannabinoids) from industrial hemp is federally legal (recall that the product must contain less than 0.3 percent THC) and CBD (and other cannabinoids) from marijuana must be purchased in a medical marijuana dispensary. When obtaining your ingredients, always ensure you're using a high-quality source. Also make sure that you're not overstating what your products can do. That is, do not make "drug claims" regarding your skincare product, which is a cosmetic, not a drug.

THERAPEUTIC ACTIONS—PHYSICAL	THERAPEUTIC ACTIONS—EMOTIONAL
warming the body, supporting circulation and movement, dispersing stagnancy, relieving aches and pains, aiding digestion, supporting the immune system, supporting the respiratory system, acting as an antibacterial and antimicrobial agent	grounding, arousing, stimulating, energizing, de-stressing, supporting inner resolve and confidence
relieving aches and pains, reducing inflammation, healing wounds, repairing tissues, supporting the immune system, supporting the respiratory system	grounding, centering, calming, sedating, strengthening confidence, aiding meditation, healing emotional wounds, reducing anxiety

Resources

It is important to source your CBD from growers/sellers you trust. We recommend doing your research and finding the right fit based on the quality and extraction method you are seeking.

To help you get started, here are a few CBD resources we like:

— Garden Om (www.gardenom.com)

— Open Book Extracts (www.openbookextracts.com)

— Hudson Hemp (www.hudsonhemp.com)

— Sun Soil (www.sunsoil.com)

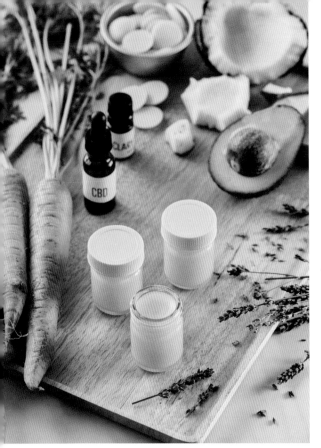

CBD BODY BUTTER

- *glass or stainless steel bowl or glass beaker*
- *double boiler (see instructions on page 198)*
- *glass or wooden stirrer*
- *4 (1-ounce) glass jars with tight-fitting lids*

- *2 tablespoons shea butter*
- *2 tablespoons cocoa butter*
- *2 tablespoons coconut oil*
- *1 tablespoon jojoba oil*
- *1 tablespoon avocado oil*
- *330 mg CBD (about 1 teaspoon CBD distillate in olive oil)*
- *70 drops lavender essential oil*
- *30 drops clary sage essential oil*
- *24 drops carrot seed essential oil*

15 MINUTES

4 (1-OUNCE) JARS

Skin dryness and itchiness usually happen when our skin struggles to retain moisture, and that's a result of a weakened skin barrier. This means that the naturally occurring oils that "glue" our skin cells together to prevent water from escaping our bodies (transepidermal water loss) and to protect us against pathogens are weak and broken, and as a result our skin feels dry and itchy.

Using a body butter rich with plant-powered ingredients like shea butter, coconut oil, jojoba oil, and avocado oil can help feed our skin the components needed to repair the weakened "glue." By also including CBD in the recipe, we can exponentially boost the healing properties of the other ingredients and power up communication with the endocannabinoid system, ultimately resulting in a more functional skin barrier.

STEPS

1. In a bowl or beaker, combine the shea butter, cocoa butter, coconut oil, jojoba oil, and avocado oil.

2. Gently place the bowl or beaker with the butter and oil mixture in the upper pot with the inch of water. Reduce the heat to low, and stir while the ingredients are melting. Continue stirring until well combined.

3. Remove the bowl or beaker that contains all the melted butters and carrier oils from the double boiler, and wipe away all the moisture and water from the outside of the bowl or beaker.

4. Add the CBD oil and essential oils to the melted mixture and stir well.

5. Slowly pour the mixture into the glass jars, cap tightly, and place immediately in the refrigerator. Refrigerate for at least 4 hours. The body butter should last for 6 months unrefrigerated. (It's best not to keep it in the fridge.)

Beauty Note!

Whenever melting shea butter in a beauty recipe, it's important to always cool it directly in the fridge. This way, the heavier molecules won't separate out and you can prevent the butter from feeling grainy.

Beauty Tip!

How to Use:

Apply liberally to dry skin as often as needed.

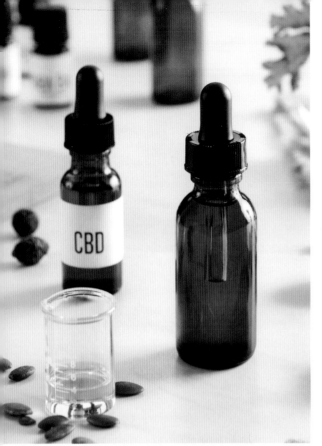

CBD FACE OIL FOR YOUTHFUL GLOW

- small glass beaker
- glass or wooden stirrer
- 1 (1-ounce) amber glass bottle with a dropper cap

- 1 tablespoon pumpkin seed oil
- 1 tablespoon argan oil
- 1½ teaspoons jojoba oil
- 1¼ teaspoons camellia seed oil
- ½ teaspoon pomegranate seed oil
- ¼ teaspoon rosehip seed oil
- 165 mg CBD (about ½ teaspoon CBD distillate in olive oil)
- 5 drops copaiba essential oil
- 4 drops frankincense essential oil
- 3 drops geranium essential oil

10 MINUTES

1 FLUID OUNCE

As we age, a lot happens to our skin. We stop producing the oils necessary to support our skin barrier function. Our hormone levels drop, reducing our skin's ability to produce the proteins needed to synthesize collagen and elastin, which give our skin its shape and stretch. By including CBD in skincare recipes intended for more mature skin, we can help the skin find new balance amid the unavoidable physiological changes of aging and, as a result, produce a more healthy, youthful appearance.

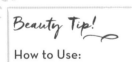

How to Use:

Apply ¼ to ½ teaspoon of the oil to your face after cleansing. Make sure to massage into your entire face and neck.

STEPS

1. In a small glass beaker, gently mix all the carrier oils and the CBD oil until fully incorporated. The color will be light orange or pink with a hint of a light brown hue; this oil will easily absorb, so don't worry about the color staining your skin.

2. Add the essential oils to the carrier oil mixture and continue stirring for about 30 seconds, until the ingredients are nicely incorporated.

3. Slowly pour the oil into the glass bottle, fasten the cap, and shake well. Your face oil is ready for use and will last for 6 months. Keep in mind that over time the aroma will intensify as the oils blossom into one another.

Beauty Note!

Face oils are a really effective and easy way to include CBD in the delivery of plant-powered components like essential fatty acids and nutrients, which are known to promote tissue repair, even out skin tone, and support resilience.

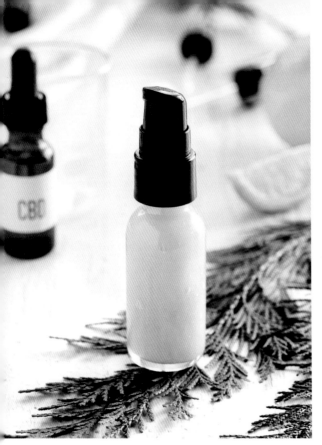

CBD ACNE SPOT GEL

- small glass or stainless steel bowl or glass beaker
- glass or wooden stirrer
- 1 (1-ounce) non-BPA plastic squeeze bottle or glass bottle with pump

- 2 tablespoons aloe vera
- 1 teaspoon tamanu oil
- 82.5 mg CBD (about ¼ teaspoon CBD distillate in olive oil)
- 10 drops cypress essential oil
- 10 drops palmarosa essential oil
- 8 drops lemon essential oil

5 MINUTES

1 FLUID OUNCE

Acne results when our skin barrier function and our skin microbiome are disrupted and bacteria settle in and cause an infection. Adding CBD to acne spot treatments can significantly speed up the healing process and refortify the skin's immunity against further infection.

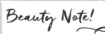

Beauty Note!

Tamanu oil has nutrients that make the oil a green color, and it may turn your gel a shade of light green.

STEPS

1. In a bowl or beaker, combine all the ingredients.
2. Vigorously stir together for about 30 seconds, ensuring all the ingredients are fully incorporated.
3. Transfer the blended product into the bottle and cap tightly. Shake well before using. The gel should last for 1 month. Keep refrigerated.

Beauty Tip!

CBD on its own does not dissolve in water. That's why you mostly see CBD as an ingredient in oil-based products like butters, balms, salves, creams, and oils. However, there are ways to incorporate it into water-based products, like this acne spot gel that uses aloe vera, a water-based ingredient.

Beauty Note!

How to Use:

Cleanse and tone your skin to create a clean surface. Apply a small drop of the acne spot treatment directly onto the affected area with your clean fingertip. Leave on and let the gel fully absorb into your skin. Repeat twice daily, or as needed.

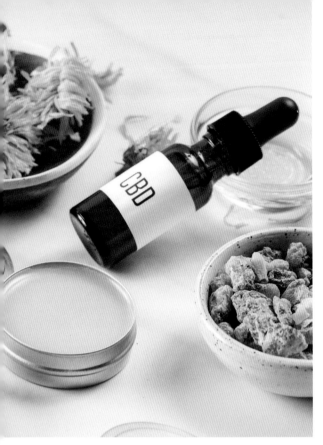

CBD PAIN RELIEF SALVE FOR INFLAMMATION AND DISCOMFORT

- *double boiler*
- *2 glass measuring pitchers*
- *glass or wooden stirrer*
- *1 (1-ounce) glass jar or metal tin with a tight-fitting lid*

- *¼ ounce organic unrefined beeswax pastilles (about 4 tablespoons)*
- *2 tablespoons arnica-infused olive oil*
- *2 tablespoons calendula-infused olive oil*
- *330 mg CBD (about 1 teaspoon CBD distillate in olive oil)*
- *7 drops lavender essential oil*
- *5 drops copaiba essential oil*
- *4 drops black pepper essential oil*
- *4 drops frankincense essential oil*
- *4 drops juniper essential oil*

2 HOURS AND

15 MINUTES

1 (1-OUNCE)

JAR OF SALVE

Inflammation is often caused by either pain or a reaction to pain. To relieve pain, we also need to reduce inflammation. We experience inflammation when our skin reacts to an external environmental stressor, like a bug bite, an allergen, or a wound. Inflammation can also result from an internal disturbance, like a strained muscle or tendon, muscle spasms, nerve distress, bruising, or injury. With this topical CBD recipe, we can engage the endocannabinoid system, soothing and calming both our internal physiology and our external reactiveness so that both can get back on track.

STEPS

1. To set up the double boiler, pour about 1 inch of water into the bottom pot and about 1 inch of water into the upper pot. Turn the heat on medium to begin warming up the water in both the lower and upper pots.

2. Once the water begins to steam a bit, add the beeswax pastilles to the first glass measuring pitcher and place it gently in the upper pot with the inch of water. Keep watch as the beeswax pastilles begin to melt.

3. While the beeswax is heating up, add the arnica- and calendula-infused oils to the second glass measuring pitcher, and mix together.

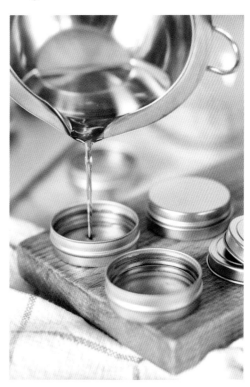

4. Once the beeswax is fully melted and no remnants of the pastilles are visible, slowly pour in the blended infused herbal oils and mix together. The melted beeswax may harden a little when the oils are poured in. If this happens, don't worry; simply use a glass or wooden stirrer to stir the mixture as it is heating to make sure the beeswax remelts and the oils incorporate completely.

5. Carefully lift the warm measuring pitcher out of the top pot of the double boiler, and dry off the outside with a towel to prevent any drips of water from getting into your glass jar or metal tin.

6. Add the CBD oil and essential oils to the melted salve and mix well.

7. Pour the warm melted salve into the container and cap tightly. Let the salve set, without shaking or mixing, until it hardens and cools. This could take a couple hours. Keep out of heat and away from direct sunlight. The salve should last for 8 to 12 months.

Beauty Note!

How to Use:

Scoop one finger of the salve into the palm of your hand and massage into areas that are feeling inflamed or uncomfortable. Carry the salve with you, and use as often as needed.

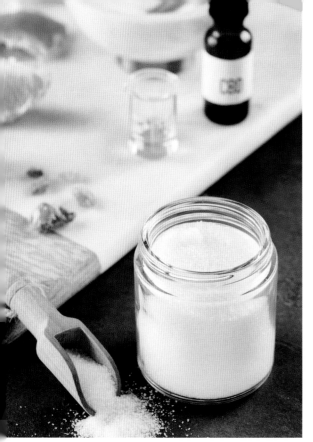

CBD BATH SALTS FOR DE-STRESSING AND RELIEVING INFLAMMATION

- *glass or stainless steel bowl*
- *1 (4-ounce) glass jar with a tight-fitting lid*

- *6 tablespoons Dead Sea salt*
- *82.5 mg CBD (about ¼ teaspoon CBD distillate in olive oil)*
- *8 drops frankincense essential oil*
- *8 drops sweet orange essential oil*
- *6 drops clary sage essential oil*

5 TO 10

MINUTES

1 (4-OUNCE)

JAR OF BATH

SALTS

Aromatic baths have a powerful effect on the body, mind, and spirit, and when we enhance the experience with CBD, our muscle aches and pains, nervous energy, and any joint swelling or inflammation can slowly melt away, offering us tremendous relief.

STEPS

1. Spoon the Dead Sea salt into a glass or stainless steel bowl.
2. Gently add the CBD oil, followed by the essential oils, and blend well.
3. Transfer the bath salts to the glass jar and cap tightly. You can use the bath salts immediately or label the jar and store it for later use (or for a gift!). If properly stored and tightly capped to avoid letting any moisture in, the bath salts can last for up to 6 months.

CBD ROLL-ON TO SOOTHE ANXIETY

- *glass measuring pitcher*
- *glass or wooden stirrer*
- *1 (0.35-ounce) glass roll-on bottle with a cap*

- *2 teaspoons jojoba oil*
- *82.5 mg CBD (about ¼ teaspoon CBD distillate in olive oil)*
- *9 drops orange essential oil*
- *8 drops lavender essential oil*
- *5 drops frankincense essential oil*

5 MINUTES

1 (0.35-OUNCE)

ROLL-ON

CBD has a powerful balancing effect on our nervous system, and for this reason it is a great ingredient to add to any recipe used to help us feel calmer and ease anxiety. Even applied in small quantities, the CBD molecules can connect with the ECS on our skin to support a balanced state of mind.

Beauty Tip!

How to Use:

Gently roll the oil blend on your temples, the back of your neck, and your scalp. Carry the roll-on with you and use as often as needed when feeling anxious.

STEPS

1. In a glass measuring pitcher, combine all the ingredients, mixing well.

2. Carefully pour the mixture into the narrow opening of the roll-on bottle. Snap the roller ball into place, cap the bottle, and shake. The roll-on should last for 6 to 8 months.

RESOURCES FOR BEAUTY BLENDING INGREDIENTS

Education

www.formulabotanica.com

www.susanmparker.com

www.theglohaus.com

Containers

www.containerandpackaging.com

www.sks-bottle.com

www.specialtybottle.com

Labels

www.onlinelabels.com

Essential Oils

www.amrita.net

www.edenbotanicals.com

www.enfleurage.com

www.erbaviva.com

www.originalswissaromatics.com

www.zayataroma.com

Carrier Oils

www.botanicinnovations.com

www.bulknaturaloils.com

www.fromnaturewithlove.com

www.jojobacompany.com

www.mountainroseherbs.com

www.soaperschoice.com

Organic Alcohol

www.organicalcohol.com

Aloe Vera Juice, Gel, and Jelly

www.lilyofthedesert.com

Antioxidants

www.fromnaturewithlove.com

www.mountainroseherbs.com

www.ohohorganic.com

www.theherbarie.com

Butters and Waxes

www.bulknaturaloils.com

www.fromnaturewithlove.com

www.glorybee.com

www.mountainroseherbs.com

www.ohohorganic.com

Clays and Salts

www.fromnaturewithlove.com

www.mountainroseherbs.com

www.naturalsourcing.com

www.realsalt.com

www.seasalt.com

Gums

www.fromnaturewithlove.com

www.theherbarie.com

Herbs

www.pacificbotanicals.com

www.starwest-botanicals.com

Hydrosols

www.edenbotanicals.com

www.fromnaturewithlove.com

www.morningmystbotanics.com

www.mountainroseherbs.com

Vegetable Glycerin

www.fromnaturewithlove.com

www.ohohorganic.com

www.mountainroseherbs.com

NOTES

Deconstructing Beauty Labels

1   Donya Fahmy, "What's in a Name? Making Sense of Ingredient Decks for Personal Care," *AllNaturalBeauty*, 2009, http://www.allnaturalbeauty.com/articles/324-whats-in-a-name-making-sense-of-ingredient-decks-for-personal-care-products-to-safeguard-your-health

2   Star Khechara and Lorraine Dallmeier, "Diploma in Organic Skincare Formulation," *Formula Botanica*, https://formulabotanica.com/diploma-in-organic-skincare-formulation/

3   Perry Romanowski, "Practical Product Development" (PowerPoint slides from lecture, Society of Cosmetic Chemists, New York City, NY, June 6, 2016), https://www.dropbox.com/s/e1dcdqj2v9n0p23/PPD-2016full-PR.pdf?dl=0

4   Ibid.

5   Jade Shutes and Amy Galper, "Botanical Body Care Certification" (course, School for Aromatic Studies, Chapel Hill, NC, November 2016).

Is Natural the Same as Organic?

1   *Merriam-Webster*, s.v. "natural," accessed November 9, 2016, https://www.merriam-webster.com/dictionary/natural

2   "Organic Regulations," *United States Department of Agriculture, Agricultural Marketing Service*, https://www.ams.usda.gov/rules-regulations/organic

How the Skin Works

1   Paul A. Kolarsick, Maria Ann Kolarsick, and Carolyn Goodwin, "Anatomy and Physiology of the Skin," *Journal of the Dermatology Nurses' Association* 3, no. 4 (2011): 203–13, doi:10.1097/JDN.0b013e3182274a98

2   Peter T. Pugliese and Zoe Diana Draelos, *Physiology of the Skin*, 3rd ed. (Carol Stream, IL: Allured Books, 2011), 1–7.

3   Ruhr-Universitaet-Bochum, "Olfactory Receptors in the Skin: Sandalwood Scent Facilitates Wound Healing, Skin Regeneration," *ScienceDaily*, July 8, 2014, https://www.sciencedaily.com/releases/2014/07/140708092555.htm

4   Jan Kusmirek, *Liquid Sunshine: Vegetable Oils for Aromatherapy* (Glastonbury, UK: Floramicus, 2002), 73.

Plant Extracts and Whole-Plant Parts

1   Marina Kamenev, "Top Ten Aboriginal Bush Medicines," *Australian Geographic*, February 8, 2011,   http://www.australiangeographic.com.au/topics/history-culture/2011/02/top-10-aboriginal-bush-medicines

2   Jan Kusmirek, *Liquid Sunshine: Vegetable Oils for Aromatherapy* (Glastonbury, UK: Floramicus, 2002), 9.

3   Kurt Schnaubelt, *The Healing Intelligence of Essential Oils: The Science of Advanced Aromatherapy* (Rochester, VT: Healing Arts Press, 2011), 14.

Beauty Ingredient Charts: Carrier Oils

1   Jan Kusmirek, *Liquid Sunshine: Vegetable Oils for Aromatherapy* (Glastonbury, UK: Floramicus, 2002), 9.

Beauty Ingredient Charts: Herbal Infusions

1   "How to Make Macerated Oils," *Formula Botanica*, http://formulabotanica.com/how-to-make-macerated-oils/

Beauty Ingredient Charts: Hydrosols

1   Ann Harman, *Harvest to Hydrosol* (Northport, WA: IAG Botanics, 2015), 5.

2   "What Are Hydrosols?," *Hydrosol World*, http://www.hydrosolworld.com/what-are-hydrosols/

Beauty Ingredient Charts: Butters

1   Jan Kusmirek, *Liquid Sunshine: Vegetable Oils for Aromatherapy* (Glastonbury, UK: Floramicus, 2002), 58–70.

2   "Processing Edible Oils," *Penn State Extension*, http://www.extension.psu.edu/natural-resources/energy/field-crops/fact-sheets/processing-edible-oils

3   Ibid.

4   "Processing and Refining Edible Oils," chap. 5 in *Fats and Oils in Human Nutrition, Food and Agriculture Organization of the United Nations*, 1994, http://www.fao.org/docrep/v4700e/v4700e0a.htm

5   "Processing Edible Oils," *Penn State Extension*.

What You Need in Your Beauty Formulation Kitchen

1   Richard C. Thompson et al., "Plastics, the Environment and Human Health: Current Consensus and Future Trends," *Philosophical Transactions of the Royal Society B: Biological Sciences* 364, no. 1526 (2009): 2153–66, doi:10.1098/rstb.2009.0053

2   Hui Gao et al., "Bisphenol A and Hormone-Associated Cancers: Current Progress and Perspectives," *Medicine* 94, no. 1 (2015): e211, doi:10.1097/MD.0000000000000211

3   "Reviews of 27 Preservatives," *Making Skincare*, http://www.makingskincare.com/preservatives

Facial Care

1   Samantha Faragalli, "Do You Actually Need to Wash Your Face in the Morning?" *InStyle*, September 13, 2015, http://www.instyle.com/news/washing-face-in-morning-necessary

2   Ibid.

3   "Almond Milk: Good for Your Skin?" *FitDay*, http://www.fitday.com/fitness-articles/nutrition/healthy-eating/almond-milk-good-for-your-skin.html

4   Elena Conis, "Poring Over Facts About Milk: Cow's, Goat's, Soy, Almond, Rice and Hemp," *Los Angeles*

Times, October 19, 2009, http://articles.latimes.com/2009/oct/19/health/he-milk19/3

5   Jade Shutes, "Aromatic Applications for the Skin" (course, School for Aromatic Studies, Seattle, WA, 1995).

6   Shannon Romanowski, "What Do Enzymes Do for Your Skin?" *Self*, February 1, 2012, http://www.self.com/flash/beauty-blog/2012/02/are-enzymes-good-for-skin/

7   The Human Microbiome Project Consortium, "Structure, Function and Diversity of the Healthy Human Microbiome," *Nature* 486, no. 7402 (2012): 207–14, doi:10.1038/nature11234

8   Anna Azvolinsky, "Birth of the Skin Microbiome," *The Scientist*, November 17, 2015, http://www.the-scientist.com/?articles.view/articleNo/44488/title/Birth-of-the-Skin-Microbiome/

9   Yiyin Erin Chen and Hensin Tsao, "The Skin Microbiome: Current Perspectives and Future Challenges," *Journal of the American Academy of Dermatology* 69, no. 1 (2013): 143–55, doi:10.1016/j.jaad.2013.01.016

10 "Our Research," *Mother Dirt*, http://www.motherdirt.com/our-research&s=n

11 Chris Kresser, "Skin Microbiota and Your Health," *Chris Kresser* (blog,) May 3, 2016, http://www.chriskresser.com/skin-microbiota-and-your-health/

12 Kristin Collins Jackson, "The Strawberry Benefits for Skin Are Even Sweeter Than You'd Imagined," *Bustle*, April 23, 2015, https://www.bustle.com/articles/76386-the-strawberry-benefits-for-skin-are-even-sweeter-than-youd-imagined

13 Saint Louis University, "Treating Acne: Two Different Acid Peels Are Both Effective, Study Finds," *Science-Daily*, February 7, 2008, http://www.sciencedaily.com/releases/2008/02/080206121508.htm

14 "Understanding Acne Treatment," *WebMD*, http://www.webmd.com/skin-problems-and-treatments/acne/understanding-acne-treatment#1

15 Israel Zeligman, "Topical Chlorophyll Therapy in the Dermatoses," *Journal of Investigative Dermatology* 13, no. 3 (1949): 111–13, doi:10.1038/jid.1949.75

16 D. Weir and K. L. Farley, "Relative Delivery Efficiency and Convenience of Spray and Ointment Formulations of Papain/Urea/Chlorophyllin Enzymatic Wound Therapies," abstract, *Journal of Wound, Ostomy and Continence Nursing* 33, no. 5 (2006): 482–90, http://www.ncbi.nlm.nih.gov/pubmed/17133135; and Y. L. Zhang et al., "The Protective Effect of Chlorophyllin Against Oxidative Damage and Its Mechanism," abstract, *Zhonghua Nei Ke Za Zhi* 51, no. 6 (2012): 466–70, http://www.ncbi.nlm.nih.gov/pubmed/22943759

17 C. Antille et al., "Topical Beta-carotene Is Converted to Retinyl Esters in Human Skin Ex Vivo and Mouse Skin In Vivo," abstract, *Experimental Dermatology* 13, no. 9 (2004): 558–61, http://www.ncbi.nlm.nih.gov/pubmed/15335356

18 Theodore L. Sourkes, "The Discovery and Early History of Carotene," *Bulletin for the History of Chemistry* 34, no. 1 (2009): 32–38, http://www.scs.illinois.edu/~mainzv/HIST/bulletin_open_access/v34-1/v34-1%20p32-38.pdf

19 "Vitamin A Fact Sheet for Health Professionals," *U.S. Department of Health and Human Services, National Institutes of Health, Office of Dietary Supplements*, http://www.ods.od.nih.gov/factsheets/VitaminA-HealthProfessional/

20 Christian Nordqvist, "What Is Beta-carotene? What Are the Benefits of Beta-carotene?" *Medical News Today*, last modified October 26, 2016, http://www.medicalnewstoday.com/articles/252758.php

21 "Opinion on Vitamin A," *European Commission, Scientific Committee on Consumer Safety*, last modified December 23, 2016, http://www.ec.europa.eu/health/scientific_committees/consumer_safety/docs/sccs_o_199.pdf

22 "NTP Technical Report on the Photococarcinogenesis Study of Retinoic Acid and Retinyl Palmitate," *U. S. Department of Health and Human Services, National Institutes of Health, Public Health Services*, August 2012, http://www.ntp.niehs.nih.gov/ntp/htdocs/lt_rpts/tr568_508.pdf

23   "13 Magical Benefits of Shea Butter for Skin, Hair and Health," *MJ Celebrity Magazine*, http://www.mjemag-azine.com/13-magical-benefits-of-shea-butter-for-skin-hair-and-health/

24   Toshihiro Akihisa et al., "Anti-inflammatory and Chemopreventive Effects of Triterpene Cinnamates and Acetates from Shea Fat," *Journal of Oleo Science* 59, no. 6 (2010): 273–80, doi:10.5650/jos.59.273

25   Elizabeth Siegel, "Can You Use Coconut Oil as Makeup Remover?" *Allure*, March 12, 2015, http://www.allure.com/story/coconut-oil-makeup-remover

26   "The Science Behind the Health Benefits of Steam Showers," *Mr. Steam* (blog), July 6, 2016, http://blog.mrsteam.com/archive/the-science-behind-the-health-benefits-of-steam-showers

27   *Wikipedia*, s.v. "Aloe vera," accessed November 27, 2016, https://en.wikipedia.org/w/index.php?title=Aloe_vera&oldid=751718067

28   Amar Surjushe, Resham Vasani, and D. G. Saple, "Aloe Vera: A Short Review," *Indian Journal of Dermatology* 53, no. 4 (2008): 163–66, doi:10.4103/0019-5154.44785

29   Ibid.

30   P. Chithra, G. B. Sajithlal, and G. Chandrakasan, "Influence of Aloe Vera on Collagen Characteristics in Healing Dermal Wounds in Rats," abstract, *Molecular and Cellular Biochemistry* 181, nos. 1–2 (1998): 71–76, https://www.ncbi.nlm.nih.gov/pubmed/9562243

31   Gina Fisher, "Lip Moisturizers 101," *How Stuff Works*, August 20, 2009, http://health.howstuffworks.com/skin-care/lip-care/tips/lip-moisturizers2.htm

32   Sierra Bright, "13 Amazing Health & Beauty Benefits of Cocoa Butter," *Natural Living Ideas*, January 21, 2016, http://www.naturallivingideas.com/13-amazing-benefits-cocoa-butter/

Hair Care

1   Lalitha Priyanka Dwarampudi et al., "Antipsoriatic Activity and Cytotoxicity of Ethanolic Extract of *Nigella sativa* Seeds," *Pharmacognosy Magazine* 8, no. 32 (2012): 268–72, doi:10.4103/0973-1296.103650

2   Paige Padgett, "Is Broccoli Seed Oil All Over Your Hair and Face Yet? (Because It Totally Should Be)," *Organic Authority*, July 14, 2016, http://www.organicauthority.com/is-broccoli-seed-oil-all-over-your-hair-face

3   Diane Mary, "4 Ways Broccoli Will Help Your Curly Hair Journey," *Naturally Curly*, May 18, 2015, http://www.naturallycurly.com/curlreading/home/4-ways-broccoli-will-help-your-curly-hair-journey/

Body Care

1   Marco Harari and Jashovam Shani, "Demographic Evaluation of Successful Antipsoriatic Climatotherapy at the Dead Sea (Israel) DMZ Clinic," *International Journal of Dermatology* 36, no. 4 (1997): 304–5. doi:10.1046/j.1365-4362.1997.00204.x. See also *Wikipedia*, s.v. "Dead Sea salt," https://en.wikipedia.org/wiki/Dead_Sea_salt#cite_note-creakyjoints-5

2   Laurice Maruek, "Dead Sea Salt vs. Epsom Salt," *Livestrong*, last modified January 9, 2014, http://www.livestrong.com/article/248504-dead-sea-salt-vs-epsom-salt/

3   J. Sharad, "Glycolic Acid Peel Therapy—a Current Review," *Clinical, Cosmetic and Investigational Dermatology* 6 (2013), 281–88, doi:10.2147/CCID.S34029

4   S. Montserrat-de la Paz et al., "Hemp (*Cannabis sativa* L.) Seed Oil: Analytical and Phytochemical Characterization of the Unsaponifiable Fraction," *Journal of Agricultural and Food Chemistry* 62, no. 5 (2014): 1105–10, doi:10.1021/jf404278q

5   Ehrhardt Proksch et al., "Bathing in a Magnesium-Rich Dead Sea Salt Solution Improves Skin Barrier Func-

tion, Enhances Skin Hydration, and Reduces Inflammation in Atopic Dry Skin," *International Journal of Dermatology* 44, no. 2 (2005): 151–57, doi:10.1111/j.1365-4632.2005.02079.x

6   Joi A. Nichols and Santosh K. Katiyar, "Skin Photoprotection by Natural Polyphenols: Anti-inflammatory, Antioxidant and DNA Repair Mechanisms," *Archives of Dermatological Research* 302, no. 2 (2010): 71, doi:10.1007/s00403-009-1001-3

7   P. Gasser et al., "Cocoa Polyphenols and Their Influence on Parameters Involved in *Ex Vivo* Skin Restructuring," *International Journal of Cosmetic Science* 30, no. 5 (2008): 339–45. doi:10.1111/j.1468-2494.2008.00457.x

8   Zoe Diana Draelos and Peter T. Pugliese, *Physiology of the Skin*, 3rd ed. (Carol Stream, IL: Allured Books, 2011), 33–36.

Personal Care

1   Janet Raloff, "Cinnamon Cleans the Breath," *Science News*, May 20, 2004, https://www.sciencenews.org/blog/food-thought/cinnamon-cleans-breath

2   L. Lakhdar et al., "Antibacterial Activity of Essential Oils Against Periodontal Pathogens: A Qualitative Systematic Review," abstract, *Odonto-stomatologie Tropicale* 35, no. 140 (2012): 38–46, https://www.ncbi.nlm.nih.gov/pubmed/23513511

3   Edward Group, "Why You Should Use Aluminum-Free Deodorant," *Global Healing Center*, last modified June 8, 2015, http://www.globalhealingcenter.com/natural-health/why-you-should-use-aluminum-free-deodorant/#2; and P. D. Darbre, "Aluminum, Antiperspirants and Breast Cancer," *Journal of Inorganic Biochemistry* 99, no. 9 (2005): 1912–19, doi:10.1016/j.jinorgbio.2005.06.001

4   "Concern over Deodorant Chemicals," *BBC News*, January 11, 2004, http://news.bbc.co.uk/2/hi/health/3383393.stm

5   Joseph Mercola, "Triclosan: The Soap Ingredient You Should Never Use—But 75% of Households Do," *Mercola*, August 29, 2012, http://articles.mercola.com/sites/articles/archive/2012/08/29/triclosan-in-personal-care-products.aspx

6   "Handwashing: Clean Hands Save Lives," *Centers for Disease Control and Prevention (CDC)*, last modified February 22, 2016, http://www.cdc.gov/handwashing/show-me-the-science-hand-sanitizer.html

GLOSSARY

Absolute: An aromatic substance produced using solvent extraction.

Acid mantle: The film that coats the outermost layer of our skin and supports its barrier function and immunity.

Analgesic: A substance that helps relieve or reduce pain.

Antibacterial: A substance that destroys bacteria.

Antidepressant: A substance that relieves or reduces depression.

Antifungal: A substance that destroys fungus or reduces or inhibits fungal growth.

Anti-inflammatory: A substance that reduces or relieves inflammation.

Antimicrobial: A substance that destroys or resists microbial pathogens.

Antioxidant: A substance or molecule that is thought to protect body cells from the damaging effects of oxidation, a chemical reaction that produces free radicals leading to damaged cells.

Antiperspirant: A substance that reduces excessive sweating.

Antiseptic: A substance that destroys or prevents the growth of microbes that could be harmful.

Antispasmodic: A substance that relieves muscular spasms.

Aphrodisiac: A substance that increases sexual stimulation and excitement.

Aromatherapy: A complementary and alternative care modality that centers on the holistic, olfactory, and therapeutic application of essential oils (see *Essential oil*) to support, enhance, and balance the physical, emotional, mental, and spiritual health of the individual.

Astringent: A substance that causes cells to shrink, contract, or tighten.

Balm: An ointment made with beeswax, vegetable and/or herbal oils, butters, and essential oils that is used to soothe skin and promote healing.

Carrier oil: A base oil used in health and beauty formulations to help dilute essential oils and "carry" them into the skin from an external application so the body can benefit from the essential oils' therapeutic properties. Carrier oils are typically derived from nuts or seeds. They possess their own spectrum of nutrients, including vitamins.

Clay: A naturally occurring substance from the earth that is used to help absorb excess oil and remove toxins and dirt from the skin.

CO_2 extraction: The method by which liquid CO_2 is used as a solvent to extract medicinal and aromatic constituents from plant materials.

Cold pressing: A high-pressure pressing method used to extract the essential oils from citrus peels.

Collagen: A complex long-chain protein that is tough and does not stretch. Skin manufactures these proteins in the dermis to help the skin keep its shape.

Deodorant: A substance that reduces or removes unpleasant body odor.

Detoxifier: A substance that supports the body's innate ability to remove excess toxic substances from the body.

Diffusion: The process of dispersing essential oils so that their natural aroma fills a room or an area.

Dilution: Diluting the potency of essential oils by blending them with a carrier, such as vegetable oils, herbal oils, butters, spray mists, and gels.

Disinfectant: A substance that destroys bacteria and pathogenic microbes.

Distillation: The method by which essential oils are extracted from plant materials using steam.

Elasticin: A protein component of fibers found in the dermis layer of the skin that provides the skin with its elasticity.

Emollient: A substance that has the effect of softening or soothing the skin.

Enfleurage: A method of extracting aromatic substances from plant material using solid (animal) fats, so that the fats are imbued with the plant's scent.

Essential oil: A highly complex molecular compound derived from the steam distillation of various aromatic plant materials like leaves, flowers, roots, seeds, wood, and roots, or the mechanical pressing of citrus rinds. Essential oils are extremely volatile and do not dissolve in water.

Exfoliation: The application of natural ingredients (such as salt, sugar, etc.) to remove dead skin cells and other debris from the surface of the skin.

Fatty acids: Constituents of vegetable oils that are essential to cellular health and stability.

Herbal oils: Vegetable oils that have been infused with medicinal herbs.

Hormonal balancer: A substance that helps balance the endocrine system.

Hydrosol: A water by-product of the steam distillation process of plant materials that contains trace amounts of the water-soluble molecules of the essential oils of the plant materials that were distilled.

Immune enhancer: A substance that supports the immune system.

Insecticide: A substance that kills or wards off insects.

Mucolytic: A substance that dissolves mucus or helps break it down so it can be released from the body more easily. It may also provide a drying effect when there is overproduction of mucus.

Neat: Refers to the act of applying an essential oil directly onto the skin without a carrier oil to dilute it.

Olfaction: The sense of smell.

Orifice reducer: A small piece of specially shaped plastic that is inserted into the neck of a glass bottle used to dispense essential oils, usually in 5 ml to 10 ml glass bottles. This small plastic piece actually reduces the amount of air that naturally circulates into the bottle and may subsequently prevent the highly volatile essential oil from oxidizing too rapidly. An orifice reducer also offers a safe way to dispense the essential oil in the form of drops. When the bottle is carefully tilted on its side, essential oil can flow through the tiny opening of the orifice reducer and be dispensed in measured drops.

Pipette: A slender disposable plastic measuring device used to transfer small quantities of liquid. It is typically used in aromatherapy to dispense essential oils drop by drop.

Salve: An ointment made with beeswax, vegetable and/or herbal oils, and essential oils that is used to soothe skin and promote healing.

Sebum: An oily substance naturally produced by the oil glands (sebaceous glands) below the skin surface.

Sedative: A substance that calms and soothes the central nervous system.

Solvent extraction: The method by which a petrochemical substance like hexane is used to extract the aromatic constituents from aromatic plant materials.

Synergy: The working together of three or more essential oils to bolster their therapeutic effectiveness as a blended formulation, as compared to their individual effects.

Toner: A substance that causes the contraction of body tissues. In beauty care, a toner is often used to help remove makeup, dirt, or remnants of soap or cleanser from the surface of the skin to prepare it to accept nourishing skin products.

Toxin: A substance that is harmful to the health of the body, mind, and environment.

USP: The US Pharmacopeial Convention (USP) is a scientific nonprofit organization that sets standards for the identity, strength, quality, and purity of medicines, food ingredients, and dietary supplements manufactured, distributed, and consumed worldwide.

Viscosity: The thickness of a fluid.

Volatility: The ability of an essential oil to evaporate or vaporize.

INDEX

RECIPE INDEX

ACKNOWLEDGMENTS

Amy's Acknowledgments

Working on any project involves a great deal of discipline and hard work. And yet, despite the tremendous effort and dedication, there is never a guarantee of the outcome. In the end, whether or not it works out is beyond our control.

I want to gratefully acknowledge all the people whose incredible hard work and dedication contributed to making this project a reality. But my deepest gratitude is to the One who is controlling it all and ultimately made it all happen.

Next, I'd like to thank my shining coauthor, Christina, who sought me out with the idea for this book (for which I am deeply honored) and throughout the process kept me focused and on point with her remarkable attention to detail and endless positivity. She was also responsible for finding our incredibly talented photographer, Cayla Zahoran, who created high art out of our wild array of kitchen tools and plant-based ingredients and made this book so very beautiful. And of course, a huge thanks to the team at BenBella Books and our extraordinary editor, Vy Tran, and Lucas Hunt, our book agent from Orchard Strategies.

I've been blessed with having had the opportunity to learn from many outstanding teachers in my life. Thank you, Joyce Piven and her late husband, Byrne; Sam Berlind; and Gay Timmons.

For many years I owned one of the first USDA-certified organic aromatherapy brands, called Buddha Nose, which received many accolades and awards. I want to thank the thousands of customers who purchased and supported that business over the years because they are an instrumental part of the trajectory that brought me to writing this book. A special thanks goes to Ethan Kahn, Beth Newburger-Schwartz, my late cousin Richard Schwartz, and my brother Josh Galper for their skilled business advice and investment in Buddha Nose.

For more recent contributions, I want to acknowledge all the students who have passed through the doors of my school, the New York Institute of Aromatherapy, and whom I have had the honor of teaching; their passion, curiosity, and enthusiasm have inspired me beyond words. In particular, I want to thank Natalya Fisher, whom I first met as my student and then hired as my assistant; she has helped me in more ways than I can ever count. Other students whose dedication I want to acknowledge are Binu Jacob and Yueyu Chen, who put in extra hours washing dishes, moving tables, and assisting at the photo shoot, while making sure things were running smoothly back at the school so I didn't have to worry.

I am also grateful to Shira Jayson, whom I mentored during the writing of this book, and Amandine Peter, one of the teachers at the New York Institute of Aromatherapy. Both spent many hours testing out all our recipes to make sure everything came out right. Other staff and faculty at the school whose dedication, passion, and presence have been especially meaningful to me include Amy Anthony, Fernanda Menegassi-Lojac, Elisabeth Vlasic, and the sweet and dedicated Celeste Knopf. And a very special thank-you goes to my 2016 summer intern from NYU, Jade Gardner, who ran around New York City doing every imaginable errand to ensure all the props for the photo shoot were in place and who worked tirelessly during the shoot, washing dishes and keeping the set clean.

Additional props for the photo shoot were supplied by Katharine L'Heureux of Kahina Giving Beauty, who lent us precious argan nuts direct from Morocco; Brian Morris from the Jojoba Company, who shared his treasured jojoba seeds; and my former student Salami A. Moyosore from Nigeria, who shipped a tub of raw shea butter directly from her family plantation and business called Organic Shoppe Nigeria. We also were fortunate to borrow both Natalya Fisher's and Raffaela P. Vergata's gorgeous handcrafted ceramics.

My family, of course, has always been there for me. I want to give special thanks to my two wonderful brothers, Adam and Josh; my angel of a mother-in-law, Donna; and Jackie, one of my sisters-in-law, who, when the idea for my school was just a glimmer, generously gifted me with my trusted KitchenAid mixer, now immortalized in the book.

And finally, I thank my parents, who gave me this miraculous life and who have always loved and supported me. My father, who always believed I would write a book someday, instilled in me a love of the written word.

But the one person to whom this book is dedicated is my husband, Stephen, who on his quest for the truth has helped bring me closer.

Christina's Acknowledgments

Writing this book has been an incredible journey, and one that could not have been possible without the support, encouragement, and love of so many people in my life.

First, my gifted teacher and coauthor, Amy, opened my eyes to aromatherapy and the art and science of plant-based medicine. She is seasoned in her craft and deeply intelligent; I am so honored to have had this opportunity to work with her.

Next, this book would not have been as compelling without the artistic eye and dazzling talent of our beloved photographer, Cayla Zahoran. Her styling, attention to detail, and creative vision transformed our ideas into visions of beauty.

I am also so deeply grateful for the talented team at BenBella Books. Thank you to our devoted and talented editor, Vy Tran, who shaped this book into what it is today; to our publisher, Glenn Yeffeth, who believed in *Plant-Powered Beauty* when it was just a seedling of an idea; and to Sarah Avinger, Jennifer Canzoneri, Adrienne

313

Lang, Alicia Kania, Monica Lowry, Heather Butterfield, and everyone at BenBella who has worked tirelessly to make this happen.

I am indebted to the agent on this book, Lucas Hunt, a trusted friend and colleague.

I subscribe to the belief that "it takes a village" to accomplish any major life task and therefore wish to also thank friends and family who were so supportive during this process. I am highlighting a few of you here, but what follows is by no means exhaustive.

Thank you to my loving and heroic husband, Simon Van Booy, and my creative and sweet daughter, Madeleine, for her endless ideas and encouragement.

I would not be in a position to write this book had it not been for my supportive parents, who are pillars of strength in my life. Thank you to Wendy Paton for her creativity and endless energy, and Jon Paton for his wisdom and devotion. And thank you to Rejean Daigneault for teaching me the value of commitment and hard work, and Evelyn Vernet Lehman for her positive spirit.

I also wish to thank the following friends and family: Vimi Bhatia, Joan and Stephen Booy, Darren Booy, Maria Christodoulou, Danielle Daigneault, Linda and Stanley Gratt, Rebecca and David Gromet, Jaclyn Inglis, Carrie Kania, Paul and Ronni Knapp, David Knapp, Aaron Malkin, Heather and David Murray, Dorit Matthews and Karl Fought, Dean and Yana Paton, Wes Paton, Alisa Schierman and Sid Horn, Christina and Matthew Wolpers, and Heidi Waintrub and Stefano Marchiaro.

I would like to make a special note in honor of my late maternal grandfather, Bert Knapp, who opened my heart to creativity with his endless stories and adventures, and my cherished maternal grandmother, Annette, who is a living example (at ninety-eight) that healthy choices can have a profound impact on wellness and longevity.

I would also like to mention my paternal grandparents, Marie-Jeanne and Laurent

Daigneault, who were lifelong farmers in Quebec, Canada. They dedicated their lives to cultivating plant life on their beautiful orchard in Rougemont, Quebec, and left me with an appreciation for nature and a love of botanicals.

During the writing of this book, in the summer of 2016, I had the great fortune to meet Wolfgang and Sabine Egger and spend time on their magical estate in Deià, Spain. Due to their kind hospitality, I spent several summer days immersed in nature, discovering exotic plant life. This experience helped inspire some of the beauty recipes found in this book.

I am also grateful to Caprice by Sophie, where I wrote and edited many portions of this book.

Also, a special note of thanks to Dr. Doni Wilson, my naturopathic doctor, who introduced me to natural wellness approaches. This led me down a path to discover aromatherapy, and for that gift I am forever grateful.

Finally, I would like to thank the Ariane de Rothschild Foundation for the incredible opportunity to participate in their program as a 2017 fellow.

ABOUT THE AUTHORS

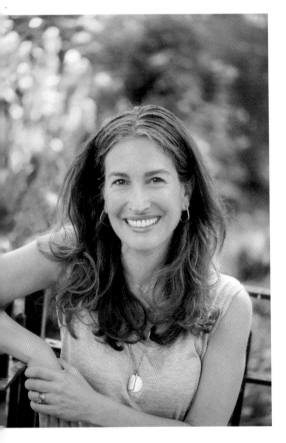

Amy Galper, BA, MA, Dipl. AT

Amy Galper is the Executive Director and Founder of New York Institute of Aromatherapy. She is a nationally celebrated advocate, entrepreneur, formulator, and consultant in organic beauty and wellness.

She is a pioneer in the field and created the award-winning, yoga-inspired line of body care products called Buddha Nose, one of the first organic brands to create national awareness of the need for toxin-free beauty and body care products. Amy also produced a series of interactive pop-up shops called "The Yoga Beauty Bar" to celebrate artisan organic beauty brands while educating women to make more conscious beauty choices.

Amy has appeared as a featured speaker at the Indie Beauty Expo, Women in Flavor & Fragrance Conference, and EcoSessions. She has been a guest lecturer at New York University and NSU College of Pharmacy and is a member of the Visiting Faculty at Arbor Vitae School of Traditional Herbalism in New York City. Amy has also been featured in dozens of top media outlets including *Cosmopolitan*, *The Dr. Oz Show*, *Prevention*, *Well+Good*, *People*, *Allure*, Refinery29, mindbodygreen, FOX NEWS, and CUNY TV.

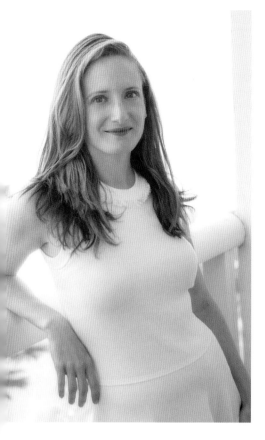

Christina Daigneault, ESQ.

Christina Daigneault is an attorney and award-winning public relations executive. She discovered the benefits of plant-based medicine and natural beauty through her work representing innovative brands and experts, which led her to earn a certification in aromatherapy from the New York Institute of Aromatherapy, where she met her coauthor.

Christina is passionate about sharing the ancient wisdom of plant-based ingredients for health and beauty. She hosts beauty blending workshops at wellness destinations around the United States and has been featured in media outlets including the *New York Times*, NBC News, Healthline, Beauty Independent, *Glamour*, mindbodygreen, and Well+Good.

Christina lives in Brooklyn, New York, with her husband and daughter.

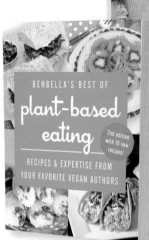
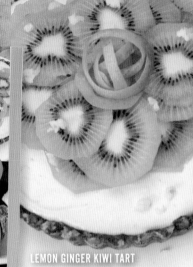
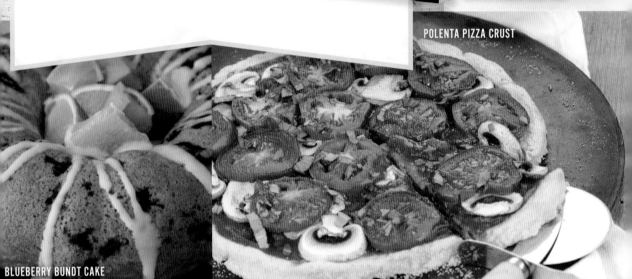